Terry—
thank you for your
service — we will
miss you in the
book —
Barbara

SIX-MONTH
CHRYSALIS

Stories, insights, and lessons from two decades
of music therapy internship experiences.

D1738196

Compiled by:
Sarah R. Sendlbeck

Edited by:
Barbara Reuer, PhD, LPMT, MT-BC

Questions? Comments?

Please feel free to contact:
> Barbara Reuer, PhD, LPMT, MT-BC
> 10455 Sorrento Valley Rd., Ste. 202
> San Diego, CA 92121
> (858) 457- 2201
> breuer@musicworxinc.com
> www.musicworxinc.com

Disclosure
For the privacy and confidentiality of our clients, all names and likenesses have been changed or removed.

"The butterfly counts not months but moments, and has time enough."

—Rabindranath Tagore

This book is dedicated to all the patients and their families whose lives were touched by music therapy over the past decades.

FOREWORD
Barbara Reuer, PhD, LPMT, MT-BC

For decades, I have proudly watched interns cycle in and out of the MusicWorx internship that I established in 1997. Collaborating with so many talented and aspiring music therapists has been a truly humbling learning experience for me as a practicing professional and mentor.

This Chrysalis is a compilation of amazing moments in music therapy transpiring over two decades in the MusicWorx internship. A unique factor of this text is that the reader will find a wide variety of settings represented in these patient highlights: from hospitals to hospice facilities, schools to substance abuse clinics, and classrooms to community centers.

We, at MusicWorx, hope that this book is as informative and enlightening to students, music therapists, and all readers as it was for the interns who engaged and learned from the experiences that they have shared here! Special thanks to all my former interns who are pioneering the field of music therapy, wherever you may be, and to the future of music therapy, the students: we salute you!

ACKNOWLEDGEMENTS

The notorious interns: thank you for your hard work during your own "six-month chrysalis" and for sharing these intimate moments and greatest "aha!" moments, which we captured and archived in this work. Esra Dalfidan, Maya Marom, Michelle Sanford, Michelle Lazar, Alex Babani, Mary Claire Mahoney, Jay Jay Lim, Traci McCune, Stella Cho, Domonique Kinney, Michelle Carlson, Susan Doering, Lara Hangebrauck, Deb Cowan, Julie Verriest, Angela Neve, Carmen Abundez, Blythe LaGasse, Melody Schwantes, Tara Dutcher, Nicole Koetting, Nozomi Nagasaka, Amy Miller, Julie Guy, Jeremy Jensen, Tricia Turner, Karen Greene, Ryoko Fukagawa, Alfonso de la Espriella, Sophia (Mary) Morreale, Theresa Camilli, Kimberly Sena Moore, Lindsay Demers, Courtney Baughman, Meridith Lager, Darci Fontenot, Elizabeth Espinoza, Shaina Pugh, Christine Giannini, Abbey Dvorak, Rachelle Norman, Davida Price, Sarah Krage, Tony Ollerton, Anna Cafazza McChesney, Rebecca Riley Olin, Kathryn Fulton, Kyle Lueken, Cynthia Tate, Ally (Jaewon) Yoon, Mutsumi Abiru, Destiny Aarone, Trina Rainey, Peggy Schaefer, Rebecca Pfeifer, Bren Yule, Chelsea Davis, Wendy Krueger, Shabnam Cyrus Mockon, Elizabeth Durrett, Veronica May, Juliana Rocha, Sara Al-Doory, Lindsey Stradt-Wilhelm, Tiffany Wyndham, Mary Altom, Katie Suddarth, Jania Isaac, Alexandra Field, Jessica Rushing, Rachel Gant, Noelle Pederson, Summer Mencher, Kymberly Tindall, Noriko Ujiie, Dayna Koehn, Leslie Jones, Tim Ringgold, Amy Andrews, Sam Brodsgaard, Rachel Kupper, Becky Human, Michael Plunkett, Allison Swain, Meryl Barns, Allyson

Moody, Rebekah Sullivan, Jey Eunyong Jang, Rebecca Vaudreuil, Anna Mitchell, Alaina Prior, Stephanie Kuester, Bahareh Moghtadaei, Desiree Gorzela, Brianna Shaffer, Christine Gallagher, Lindsay Hirata, Meredith Harvey, Julia Oh, Laura Anderson, Laura Frank, Cara Brindisi, Jennifer Spivey, Emily Paar, Carly Ramthun, Christina Whipple, Jenna Bollard, Catie Alpeter, Jessica Johnson, Audrey Lackey, Oliver Jacobson, Marlys Woods, Orion Boucher, Kristin Sjoberg, Hannah Bronson, Katie Fitch, Maya Zebley, Marielle Sheppel, Anna Smith, Amy Dunlap, Brianna Larsen, Hannah Glasson-Darling, Kristen McSorley, Esther Craven, Lindsay Tucker, Kamica King, Aida Sanchez, Mikayla Beaulieu, Derek Royce, Sara Cannon, Kelly Robertson, Hannah Andrist, Diane Garrison, Anna Andersson, Mandi Griggs, Carly Flaagan, Miranda Peyton, Michele Burns, Alex Lesser, Lindsay Zehren, Cole Eisenmenger, Allie Longworth, Katie Cox, Joe Scharnweber, Samantha Albrecht, Emily Lobeck, Annela Flores, Cory Woodrow, Sarah Folsom, Jenny Madrigal, Erik Hylan, Jordyn Shaffer, Aaron Berenson, David Burch, Tiffanie Christiansen, Whitney Hewlett, Blake Anderson, Adessa Campbell, Leah Weigel, and Marybeth Hughes.

CONTENTS

INTRODUCTION

By Sarah R. Sendlbeck

"I aspire to inspire before I expire."

–Alina Morelli

Throughout my "chrysalis" from intern to therapist, I wrote down weekly stories about my internship experiences, just like the 104 interns before me and the dozens that have gone through the internship since then. We lovingly refer to these as our "patient highlights." As you can imagine, after each intern had written one reflection every week for six months, the collection of highlights had grown extremely large. Binders upon binders burst with valuable stories on the shelves.

I reflected on my experience as a music therapy student. When I was in school, the intern world seemed so far away and so foreign. I had no idea what to expect, what types of situations I would encounter, or how I would even begin to handle them. As I looked through the stories and notes from interns before me, I thought, "These stories should be shared." I hand-selected each story that is included in this book with the hope that students, interns, new professionals, and seasoned veterans can benefit from the raw truth and beauty in each one. Let's go on a journey together: a six-month chrysalis.

Chapter 1 - The Spark

We all have those moments. Those times where you meet a new client (a stranger) and you totally hit it off. A surge of electricity runs through the room, or you wish the session could last all day. We all strive for the connection and relationship between therapist and client. It is "the spark."

Chapter 2 – Music: The Universal Language

Language is a way for humans to communicate and connect; however, it can also be a barrier at times. One beautiful aspect of music therapy is that we do not need words to communicate with our patients. The music does it for us and sometimes more deeply than any verbal exchange. Music is said to be "an understanding between human beings."

Chapter 3 - Leave Yourself at the Door

Being authentically present with patients is critical to a therapist. Being present allows us to move in the moment, be flexible if the situation dictates, and address a client's immediate needs.

Chapter 4 – Forget About It

We all have a history. Every client comes from a different background and has been shaped by their unique experiences and morals. Music therapists must separate their own beliefs from the work, view each client as an individual, and enter a session without preconceptions.

Chapter 5 - The Elevator Pitch

Every music therapist (from undergraduate student to professional) has an elevator pitch ready in their back pocket. Sometimes we encounter individuals who are curious about music therapy as a profession, do not understand the efficacy of the field, or have general questions about the modality. We gather our energy, set aside personal frustrations, and accept that advocacy and education are part of the job. Advocacy is the key to moving the field forward.

Chapter 6 - We Are Family: Support Through Music

We often provide interventions that are just as much for the family as they are for the patient. These sessions have proven to be meaningful and deep. We encourage families to interact and support one another while creating a healing environment.

Chapter 7 - Fragile Moments

Hospice, pain, illness, death: these experiences are difficult to talk about and an emotional roller coaster for the client, their families, caretakers, and music therapists. When music sets the tone, sharing in these processes can yield beautiful and touching moments for all.

Chapter 8 - Help Me, Help You: Working with Others

Interdisciplinary treatment and working with other professionals can enhance a music therapy experience or it can prove more challenging. What really matters is how we work within the situation to best serve the patient.

Chapter 9: It's Not You, It's Me: Dealing with Declines

Learning to step back and react professionally with clients who do not accept our services is not always easy. What could we have done differently to change the outcome? We are providing patients the opportunities to make decisions about what care they do and do not receive. Not everyone will want music therapy, and that is OK!

Chapter 10: I Am <u>Not</u> with the Band

A common misconception of music therapy is that we are "entertainers." This is especially difficult to handle as an intern or a new professional (especially after spending so much time, energy, and finances completing the degree program). Promoting education and advocacy helps others understand the worth of music therapy and gives meaning to the field.

Chapter 11 - Jaw Dropping: Those Exceptional Moments

"This is the reason I am a music therapist." Going to school, having bad days, or being questioned by other professionals can get you down and make you forget why you took this path. Those "wow" moments make everything worthwhile: seeing the benefits of your work in client interaction; catching the smile on a client's face; feeling the light in your heart.

Chapter 12 - The Butterfly: Spread Your Wings

We are constantly growing and changing. We go through change as students, we transform as interns, and we soar as professional music therapists. Throughout internship and professional practice, there are constant moments of development and growth. Allow yourself to accept change, embrace what you have learned, and fly far in your career.

Six-Month Chrysalis

"I feel like my experience as an intern can be compared with the stages of a butterfly. I started out as a student, a caterpillar, with a lot of book learning and little experience. I came to internship, which is kind of like a cocoon. You are surrounded and enveloped by so many experiences to help you learn and grow. Eventually, it's time for the cocoon to start breaking open. You feel more confident and almost ready to be out on your own. Just before the internship ends, the cocoon opens and out comes a butterfly— or in this case a music therapist— ready to fly on its own."

– Julie Guy, MM, MT-BC, former MusicWorx intern

CHAPTER 1 – THE SPARK

"We seek not rest but transformation. We are dancing through each other as doorways."

— Marge Piercy

A SIMPLE CONNECTION
A Patient with Rett Syndrome

I had never worked with a person who has Rett syndrome before. When I first observed the therapists working with a female patient with this diagnosis, I was amazed at the ease with which they worked and the responses they evoked. I could not imagine myself in the therapist role in this situation and was quite intimidated by the task.

I was nervous the first time I interacted with this client. I had a solid session plan with plenty of interventions to pull from, but I wondered if she would respond to me. I began slowly, using her usual greeting songs, improvising about her outfit and the music we were going to make throughout the session. The client was awake, but she seemed a bit skeptical of us as newcomers.

As we began to play music and she heard her favorite songs, she perked up and began to move her hands to play the bells. Next, I stretched her body, starting with her left side. To my surprise, she blinked "Yes" when I asked her if she wanted to stretch and she kept her eyes on mine most of the time, responding to my questions. At that point, I began to feel the energy of our session. By the end, I had connected with the client, and it seemed as if I was successful in improving her quality of life for that hour.

The client and I enjoyed our session, but had the nurse thought the interventions succeeded as well? As I prepared to leave, my worries were put to rest when the nurse shared that she felt the client had enjoyed all the music — and so had the cat! I soon realized that this was her way of saying she had enjoyed it too. I learned that gaining the trust and support of a caregiver is as important as getting it from the patient. I left feeling great, knowing I had formed a bond with the client and her nurse.

My Heart Will Go On
A Coronary Bypass Recipient

I was absolutely delighted the first time I got to be independent during my internship. My mission for that first day on my own was to make at least one meaningful connection with a patient.

I had spent the morning co-leading sessions when I received a referral for a woman who was about to be discharged from the hospital after her coronary bypass surgery. The patient had heard about music therapy and specifically requested a visit before she left the hospital. Lunch had just arrived, so I quickly checked in to see how she was feeling and to assess her musical preferences.

She was sitting up in bed with a large ruby-red heart-shaped pillow by her side. As soon as I introduced myself, before asking about her musical taste, she opened her laptop and shared her love of Native American drums. She had travelled to Australia, led drum-making workshops, spent days in sweat lodges, and walked on hot coals. This woman plainly needed a farewell meditation. I assured her that I would return with buffalo drums in the afternoon.

When I returned later that day, I came prepared with many drums, a Native American flute, and recordings of singing bowls. This would be no ordinary session. After entraining together on the drums, the patient discussed some of her experiences and as she spoke, she started to weep. "I had lost my heartbeat," she said. "Do you know how awful it is to have your heart stop for five hours while a machine keeps you alive?" Regarding our improvisation, she said, "That drum was my heartbeat."

Lessons Learned

"Stepping out of the box can lead to powerful connections and experiences. Setting an intervention for the day positively influences my perspective as a therapist."

I suggested that the patient meditate while I played the rhythm of her new heartbeat over the sound of the toning bowl. This represented her heart chakra, bringing forth the intention of life, health, and energy. Receptive to the experience, she closed her eyes, and the rhythm took over–lub-dub, lub-dub, lub-dub.

The room was alive with a quiet energy. The sound of the singing bowl filled our chests as the patient and I matched its pitch, internalizing the vibrations. She appeared to be experiencing strong emotions as her eyes brimmed with tears and she began to breathe heavily. Gradually, she relaxed and allowed the vibrations to wash over her as she hugged her ruby-red pillow.

When the sound faded away, the patient said, "That was amazing. There was no blood flowing in my artery, but while you were playing, I felt like the blood suddenly rushed through. I feel it even now." She thanked me repeatedly with gratitude that echoed the rhythm of her heartbeat— "thank you, thank you, thank you."

I thought to myself: "Mission accomplished."

THE FIRECRACKER
A Patient with Acute Lymphoblastic Leukemia

The patient was sitting up in bed, talking on the phone, with her husband at the bedside. The husband waved me in with sparkling enthusiasm and expressed his delight in receiving such a service from the hospital. As the patient finished her phone call, he introduced his wife: "This is the Firecracker," he said. "She earned that nickname the very first day I saw her, and we've been crazy about each other ever since." The Firecracker beamed at her husband with a radiant love.

The Firecracker was aptly named. A fire within her gave off a bright light to everything around her. Her beautiful smile and twinkling eyes moved me. She had filled her room with affirmations, "I am healthy!" "I am whole!" "I have joy!" "I am getting out of here!"

She explained that her chemotherapy treatment for acute lymphoblastic leukemia made green flashes when eradicating the bad cells; therefore, she'd written reminders of "green flash!" all over the room. She had even named her IV pole, "Jack," which beeped away throughout the session. We laughed, as this beeping became the solo pulse for our spontaneous song, "Call the Nurse and Gimme a Refill!"

The nurse came in to take Firecracker's vitals; her heart rate was elevated. Firecracker and her supportive husband were eager to participate in a relaxation experience. Not having a breathing script, I boldly began an improvised experience (for the first time ever). The words flowed out of me, affirming her light, appreciating the loving connection, the supportive exchange of breath, and healing process.

When the relaxation exercise ended, they opened their eyes and immediately I felt a connection with them. Extraordinary peace enveloped us.

YOU SEE MY SOUL
Long-Term Hospitalization Patient

I was working with a patient whom I had seen twice before. She was a wonderful, knowledgeable woman who speaks several languages and says she "loves all music." Each week, I learned more about her, even though she did not speak more than three or four words per session. During this session, I found how important music was to her and how it can create a powerful connection between people.

I'd discovered the previous week that German is her native language. As I began singing a German lullaby, she opened her eyes and stared at me intently. When I concluded the lullaby, she reached her hands toward me and began crying, saying, "Beautiful music, don't stop."

I sang through the lullaby several more times, and each time I concluded the song, the patient repeated, "Don't stop, don't stop." She began singing the lullaby with me, something she had never done before. Typically, she would lay with her eyes closed throughout the duration of each session.

"Did you used to sing this lullaby?" I asked.

"My mother used to sing it," she answered. She also sang it to her own children. I asked if the lullaby brought back memories for her; she nodded with tears in her

❀ LESSONS LEARNED ❀

"I am reminded each and every day of the power of music to create bonds, to create connections, and to evoke memories."

eyes, saying that the song was important to her. She began singing the lullaby once more, repeating the words to herself. I joined her and continued to sing it as she slowly fell asleep. When I got up to leave the room, she reached for my hand and held it tightly, staring at me intently. She held my hand until she slowly fell asleep once more.

That session was the most personal, raw, and emotional experience I had ever had with any human being. Music created such a connection between us; it is difficult for me to put it into words. I felt as if she had stared into my soul. The lullaby brought back such powerful memories for her that it was as if she was no longer in the room, but in another place with her mother and her children. I feel privileged to have shared such a powerful memory with her.

FIND YOUR WAVE
A Young Adult in the Surgical Intensive Care Unit

A nurse approached me to warn me about a specific referral. She described a 39-year-old man who had been doing crystal methamphetamine for five days before running his car into a tree, causing blunt chest trauma. She continued to explain that he was very anxious due to detoxifying from the drugs and asked if we could play soft soothing music for him.

When we approached his bed, he was visibly agitated with his legs restlessly moving around. He held one arm close to his chest and kept his eyes closed most of the time, occasionally opening them a sliver. I began to play the guitar (soft, slow picking) eventually joining in with my voice, matching the lullaby of the guitar. I sang "Me Ke Aloha" and then I initiated a music and imagery exercise.

As I quietly played the guitar, I talked to the patient calmly, telling him to breathe in and out, talking about the beach and the smell of the ocean, paddling out on his surfboard and looking for a wave. I looked up at his heart rate monitor and saw that his heart rate was slowly rising.

As he paddled out, reached his wave, and pushed himself up, his heart rate rose to 101. Then, as he rode the wave and I reaffirmed that he was in control, his heart rate began to decrease slowly until it reached 90. Throughout this experience, he peered at me through squinted eyes. A few times, I told him, "You're there. You're in control." Then the patient opened his eyes fully and looked right at me. He commented about the sea turtles swimming nearby.

I have never experienced music therapy with someone in this state. I was moved by the special connection that was formed between the music, the voice, and the patient. As I left, I reminded him, "Just breathe. You're in control."

REQUITED LOVE

A Man with Hodgkin's Lymphoma

A Hodgkin's lymphoma[i] patient whom I had recently seen had been in my thoughts for several days. When I first came into his room, he was standing up and his wife was lying down on his hospital bed. He happily agreed to a music therapy session, confessing that when he saw me walk by with my guitar, he hoped I would stop in.

At his request, we went out to the lobby, accompanied by his wife. I discovered that he was quite the guitarist, so I offered him my guitar to play. He declined, saying that he wanted to wait a bit. Both he and his wife are devout Christians and enjoy contemporary Christian music. The three of us sang a few of their favorites. Finally, he requested the guitar.

This patient was a wonderful musician. He played for a while, really getting into his music. He stopped and told me about the songs he had just played, all of which were his original compositions. He informed me that he had been so sick the past month that he had not been able to play and he missed it. He continued to play, sometimes stopping to explain his technique or his inspiration for a specific piece. He sang a love song for his wife that he'd written for her. The patient's love of the guitar and music was obvious and his energetic playing reflected his excitement. His wife even commented on his high energy and maintenance of activity, which had been low and inhibited for some time.

The patient finally reached his limit and returned the guitar, requesting a song that was dear to me. I sang "Besame Mucho," and the patient asked for a copy of the chords so he could play and sing it to his wife. He was scheduled to be discharged from the hospital the next day, but he asked that I come back in the morning. He and his wife hugged me, and we went our separate ways.

The next morning, his wife informed me that her husband had received a chemotherapy treatment the previous evening and had endured a rough night. Groggy and tired, he could barely stay awake to chat for the short time I was there, but he squeezed my hand, thanking me and telling me how much he had enjoyed our previous session. It was quite a contrast to the man I had met the day before. I stood in front of the elevators with a lump in my throat, moved by this client that I had come to know in such a short time.

I felt a special connection with this patient. In retrospect, I think the music helped to make that happen. Music bridges gaps between ages and cultures, puts people in a common place to share an emotion. My assessment was what this man needed the most was to play the guitar and immerse himself in the music. Music was an active, everyday part of this man's life, and he had not been able to enjoy that for a month due to his illness. Playing the guitar was the solace he needed during his difficult time.

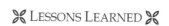

✄ LESSONS LEARNED ✄

"This experience was one in which the music was the primary therapist."

SING TO ME
End of Life with an Older Adult

Since the first session, this patient described feeling confused, anxious, and scared of not really knowing what was going to happen to him. Music therapy appeared effective in helping him release anxiety and find some peace of mind. He had also expressed appreciation of music therapy services, requesting that I come back as soon as I could arrange it.

This day, my third session with him, he was asleep when I walked into his room, so I decided to come back in about an hour. When I returned, he was still sleeping and mumbling at times, so I checked with his nurse to see if I could wake him up; she agreed to the session. I began humming a soft melody to the sound of the violin and gently touching the patient's shoulder to wake him. He opened his eyes and appeared scared at first. I explained to him that he could just relax to the sound of the music from his bed. He said that would be fine, but soon he began complaining about cramps on his feet and said he wanted to walk.

I asked the nurse to help the patient to the restroom and while he walked to the restroom, he complained about the cramps. His facial expression was tight, so I asked him to take slow deep breaths while focusing on the sound of the violin. After he got to the restroom, his facial expression was more relaxed and he was no longer complaining. As soon as he began walking back to his wheelchair, the music began playing again and he requested that we play "Shenandoah." He sang along for almost the entire song and as soon as we finished it, he began singing it a cappella on his own. At every line, his voice grew heavier with emotion and I felt like crying as I remembered talking to him previously about singing to help him feel better.

I looked at that man in the wheelchair, singing "Shenandoah," with tired eyes, a tired body, at the end of his life. I realized

Lessons Learned

"People pass through our lives, and we pass through people's lives. Each one of us has a story, something to tell, to share."

he wasn't simply singing a song; he was telling us a story. He was sharing with us part of who he was. That moment was truly a gift.

This patient made me realize how important the gift of life is to us all. I reflected on what really matters as we travel through this short 'journey of life.' Life is music, music is life, and we are all composers of our own symphony. This patient had shared part of his journey with me. And it was truly a highlight.

REMEMBERING WHAT MATTERS
Gastric Cancer Patient

I saw a cancer patient who was originally from Latin America but had moved to the United States to be with family as his health declined. During my initial session with this patient, he was passionate about music and responded to music therapy by saying, "You have no idea how you've made my heart soar."

For the next session, I noticed he looked rather despondent. He was sitting up in bed with his arms propped on his knees, his head hanging down, and his eyes closed. He smiled at me sadly when I entered. "It has not been a good day. I am feeling down," he said.

Earlier in the day, he had received morphine for his pain. At the time of my visit, he said his body was no longer in pain, but his "spirit was hurting." I played some classical pieces on guitar and hummed as he listened, often closing his eyes and moving his head in time with the music.

Seeing that he had become more emotionally stable, I invited the patient to try playing music on a kalimba (an African finger piano). He hesitantly took it and experimented and interjected self-critique, but continued after I encouraged him. After a few more minutes of experimenting, the patient noted that it was a relaxing instrument and asked if they were available for purchase, wanting his son to buy one for him.

✂ LESSONS LEARNED ✂

"During school, becoming absorbed in everything one must do to meet deadlines and stay on top of coursework can become 'all consuming.'. This experience was a fresh reminder to make time for the things that stir my passions - my wants - lest they die away."

The patient becoming fatigued, so I asked if he wanted to continue playing or rest. He requested rest, as "the medicine makes me tired." He then shared that he felt he was not honoring a promise he made to his now-deceased mother regarding pain management. She did not accept a hip replacement for a broken hip in her last year due to religious reasons. Her belief deeply affected him in a profound way. He explained that she felt the morphine was causing pain in his spirit while alleviating pain in his body.

As he was sharing this story with me, he began to cry. We discussed the important role his mother played in his life, and I stated that she sounded like a woman from whom he drew a great deal of wisdom; the patient concurred. I invited him to close his eyes and allow the music to wash over him as I improvised a relaxation exercise with humming and guitar. When I finished, the patient opened his eyes and said, "You took me to a better place." As I was preparing to leave, he said, "I feel much better. Thank you for your gift." He extended his hand to take mine in appreciation.

When everything seems to come together it is a wonderful feeling for a music therapist. Although connecting with patients is inevitable, no patient affected me as profoundly as this one. From speaking with the nursing staff, he is clearly a man who lives his life with integrity and passion. His zeal for his family and the things he loves was infectious and encouraged me to re-evaluate the areas where I have allowed the 'musts' to overshadow the 'wants.'

HUMAN CONNECTIONS
Woman Suffering Injuries from a Bilateral Fall

Upon entering her room, the patient was sitting up in her chair, with her head down. She had a blanket wrapped around her shoulders and appeared sad, yet she welcomed music therapy into her room. Her face lit up when I asked her what type of music she enjoyed. She sat up a little in her chair and slowly, carefully began to tell us stories about camping with her children and sitting around the campfire. She said, "We used to sing!"

Music held a special place in this woman's heart. To stay true to the campfire spirit, I sang, "Home on the Range."

She mustered all her strength to belt out a few phrases and words here and there, all the while having the cheeriest demeanor. Thinking hard to herself, she stumbled for her words. She then asked if we knew how to play "Amazing Grace."

Kneeling on the floor next to the patient's chair, I held her hands and sang "Amazing Grace." After the song ended, the patient nodded her head and said, "Thank you so much. People forget there is something special about music. It feels good to sing, and when you sing with others, it makes you feel connected with people. Thank you for coming to sing with me."

> **LESSONS LEARNED**
>
> *"Not only are we strumming a guitar or singing, we are connecting with a human being."*

We use a powerful tool with our patients. Not only does music bring back memories for some—a time when they were happy or sad—it also allows us as humans to connect in the present. Something as simple as singing two songs with patients and giving them something they haven't felt in a while can change their whole outlook on the day and their current situation. We are human beings first, and we all crave connections with others.

CHAPTER 1: QUESTIONS FOR GROWTH

1. Have you experienced a "wow" moment or a quote from a patient that has made you think of music therapy in a more powerful way? Explain.

2. The spark between therapist and client is what we strive for, but what does a healthy relationship between therapist and client look like? What is acceptable and what is unacceptable in a therapeutic relationship?

3. What is a personal lesson you have learned from a patient? A professional lesson?

4. As a therapist, what is an appropriate response when a patient asks you something heavy such as what was exemplified in "My Heart Will Go On," ... *"Do you know how awful it is to have your heart stop for five hours while a machine keeps you alive?"*

5. In this chapter we read about an intern who used a patient's IV monitor as a pulse/metronome for the music in the session. What is the founding principle behind this technique? What other interventions and/or exercises can you do in medical music therapy session by incorporating clients' medical devices?

6. As therapists, what can we do to build rapport with caregivers, and why is it important?

7. A few different terms and diagnoses have been used in this chapter. How many can you define?
   a) Rett Syndrome
   b) Lymphoblastic leukemia
   c) Hodgkins lymphoma
   d) Bilateral fall

CHAPTER 2 - MUSIC: THE UNIVERSAL LANGUAGE

"Music expresses feeling and thought, without language; it was below and before speech, and it is above and beyond all words."

— *Robert G. Ingersoll*

THE THREE SENSES

A Young Man who is Deaf and Blind

I saw a 14-year-old boy, blind and deaf from birth. He came into the room very stiff and agitated, so I tried doing percussive rhythms on his body. The constant drumming he received on his back and chest caught his attention. He seemed curious; his body relaxed a bit and he stayed still.

I repeated this in our next session and presented a drum for him to play. I would first take his hand and play the drum with it. I felt a real connection. After a while, he played the drum voluntarily, and I would reinforce what he had just played on his back. We got into a playful dynamic, back and forth, for about 20 to 30 seconds. It turned into a call-and-response game, and I felt we communicated nicely.

For me, that was an exciting moment. Finding a channel of communication with someone whose main channels (vision and hearing) are closed is difficult. But with the percussive experience - for a while - we spoke the same language.

GO THE EXTRA MILE

Hospice Patient with Prostate Cancer

I was always nervous before seeing patients that didn't speak English, because I felt uncomfortable not being able to communicate. This hospice patient spoke only Spanish, and I spoke English, but somehow we communicated. Before going into the room for my second visit, I reviewed some Spanish-language flashcards a couple of times so I could use basic phrases in the session. I introduced myself and asked if he would like to hear some music. He said, "Yes, that would be beautiful," and so I asked him to pick a song.

He chose "Besame Mucho" and we sang through it, continuing to several other songs. Between the songs, I conversed with him using my limited Spanish and the words from the songs we sang. We also used sign language and laughter to communicate with each other. I was in his room for 40 minutes and enjoyed every bit of it.

> ✹ LESSONS LEARNED ✹
>
> *"Remember not to be intimidated if you can't communicate verbally with a patient. Sometimes we communicate more effectively in other ways."*

This experience reminded me that if you challenge yourself, are creative, and put forth the extra effort, you could overcome language barriers and communicate. It might even be the best session all day!

LET DOWN THE WALL
A Woman's Pre-Operation Support

As I walked through the hospital hallway, I saw a woman sitting in bed with her husband beside her. He smiled and motioned for me to come inside. I quickly looked at the chart for her name and diagnosis and walked into the room.

I entered the presence of a loving but hurting couple. They had just gotten married and she was in the hospital to undergo back surgery. The surgery posed a risk of paralysis, but she was willing to take that risk because she constantly endured crippling pain and could no longer walk. I explained music therapy to the patient and her husband ~ they seemed eager to begin the session. She immediately requested that I sing her favorite song, "Amazing Grace." As I began singing, the patient sang along, crying.

I noticed that her husband looked away from her the entire time, as if he was disassociating himself from the room and the situation. When I finished singing, she continued crying, stating, "I really needed to hear that song." Her husband expressed his appreciation; however, I noticed that he did not comfort his emotional wife.

At this time, the patient's roommate requested, "With A Little Help from My Friends." As I began singing the song, both the patient and her husband began smiling and singing along as well. I noticed that they made significantly more eye contact during this song. After, they both expressed their appreciation. Her husband began talking about how he was told that he was tone deaf when he was younger and that he feels extremely self-conscious about his singing. I reassured him that the session was not about musicality or singing technique, but about the process involved and the intentions behind the music. I asked him if he could sing any song right now (without judging his own singing voice) what would it be? He responded immediately with, "I would sing a love song to my beautiful bride."

He flipped through my book and chose "I Can't Help Falling in Love with You." I began playing the song and prompted him to sing to his wife. They turned toward each other and away from me as if they were transported into a different time and place.

They sang to each other and cried until they turned toward me and indicated that they were ready to end the song and the session. The patient stated that this was the first time her husband had sung to her, and said, "This made my day." Her husband said he had never felt comfortable singing until this day.

❈ LESSONS LEARNED ❈

"Each week I experience the power of music to connect individuals, break down boundaries, and build connections"

Music enabled this couple to deeply share their thoughts, feelings, and love with each other in a new way.

Music allowed them to process their emotions and to be present with each other during a difficult time. I feel honored to have been a part of their special and intimate experience.

BRIDGING THE GAP
Ovarian Cancer Patient

I had a session with a 44-year-old Spanish-speaking woman diagnosed with ovarian cancer. I observed her in bed and alert. The entire session was conducted in Spanish because my co-therapist and I are bilingual.

We began by singing "Besame Mucho," and the patient said, "You sing so beautifully!" We asked what kind of music she enjoyed and she said, "Everything." We chose the song "Que Sera Sera," and I explained what the song meant since a majority of the song was in English. After the explanation, the patient started talking about her family, her past, and her future. She became emotional, tears flowing down her face, as she discussed her family and her fears of the unknown. Knowing that this patient was benefiting from talking to someone she trusted, we provided space for her to talk for about 10 minutes until we sang the last song, "Amazing Grace." The patient thanked us for the music and said that the music sounded "like angels."

This session reinforced that language is no barrier when music is used. The music allowed the client to openly talk about her feelings, concerns, thoughts, and hopes for the future. Many stressors in her life worried her; allowing her to talk was important. The lyrical content of our song selections were vital because they related to her needs.

SILENT APPROVAL
A Non-Verbal Former Jazz Musician

This encounter was an incredible experience for me. The patient was a 75-year-old African- American male with a brain tumor. He was a former professional jazz clarinetist who played and recorded with various jazz legends many years ago.

As much as I wanted to work with this man, I was nervous and apprehensive not only because of his level of musicianship and notoriety in the jazz world, but also because his son said the man was basically non-verbal. However, the son clearly stated that his father would let us know if he liked what we were doing by using body language and facial expressions. So many thoughts ran through my mind, like "What if I play something and he hates it," and "What if I keep playing and he can't tell me he wants me to stop?" and "Nothing I play is going to sound good because we have the keyboard and no sustain pedal." I was quite fearful about my ability to help this patient and to communicate with him without verbal responses.

We walked into the room and I introduced myself. The patient was lying in his bed with his back propped up and his wife sitting next to him. As I suspected, she agreed on jazz as the music of choice. At first, the patient was quite lethargic and difficult to read. He nodded his head slowly when we suggested the first tune. During and after the first song, he had a card held up over his face, covering everything but his eyes. I thought, "He is trying to hide his laugh." His wife lowered his hands, but his face was still difficult to read. We suggested another song, and he again nodded his head slowly. As I played and sang, I made eye contact a few times with him. He stared at me, but whether he was approving or disapproving of the music was impossible for me to determine. My thoughts were screaming, "What is he thinking? Surely he's thinking about the horrible key changes I am making."

After the third song, I closed the songbook and began to end the session. Suddenly, the patient got a distressed look on his face. It was the first time I could interpret his expression. I asked him, "Oh! You want us to stay?" He nodded. I felt a wave of warmth and relief wash over me. As we proceeded with more songs, he continued to stare into my eyes, but with each song, his eyes and facial expressions softened, and a smile came upon his face. When asked if he liked the song, he softly said, "Yes." His eyes were so intense, it felt as if they burned right into my soul, and I knew the music was bringing him just what he needed at that moment. His eyes said it all.

I had never felt so connected to a patient; which was so bizarre because there were hardly any words exchanged. I did not want to leave the room, I felt like singing to him for the rest of the night.

After the session, I poured over his chart and learned that he was a retired psychologist. I thought, "A psychologist and a professional jazz musician? What conversations we could have."

I thought back to the insecurities and anxiety I had felt when the session began. I hadn't been confident in my musical abilities or my communication skills. These fears nearly led me to end the session early, even though the patient clearly wanted to hear more. This man who played among jazz legends, a man who could barely talk. I witnessed the connection, communication, beauty and gift that music offered. Most of all, I learned that I need to let go of myself.

✖ LESSONS LEARNED ✖

"I learned in this encounter how much my own self-criticism and fears have the power to limit not just me, but others from receiving the healing gift of music. Let go of yourself."

OUT OF THE BLUE

An Older Woman in End-of-Life Care

A hospice nurse told me that she had a priority referral - a new patient whose end was nearing. I had seen this patient's roommate the previous week and she (the referred patient) had been unresponsive.

I entered the room and went over the roommate's bed first. The curtain was drawn between the women's beds for privacy. I began to softly sing composed and improvisatory songs (mostly spiritual). I kept my voice soft and low. Suddenly, I heard, "Don't keep it down on my account, I'm enjoying it," said the referred patient from the other side of the curtain. This response shocked me because the last time that I had seen her, that woman had not responded at all.

After the session ended with the first patient, I went to the other woman's side of the room. She smiled at me and asked, "Were you the one singing that beautiful music?" I replied and asked if she would enjoy any music for herself. She said, "Oh, yes please. That would be so lovely."

She told me that she is a religious woman and it meant so much to her to hear those spiritual songs. She missed going to church and felt that, for a moment during the music, she was there again. We sang through a few of her other favorites and discussed them. We talked about how she loves to speak Spanish even though she really doesn't know the language, how she hates new music and has a deep respect and love for the old tunes. She told me all about her parents and childhood, and she reminisced about the songs of her youth.

She then asked me to choose a song for her. I chose "Somewhere Over the Rainbow." As I began to sing, she said, "Who doesn't know that one? Gosh, I wish I could sing along with you." She said her voice is something that gives her a lot of trouble. I told her that even if she could not sing she could mouth the words along with me. From this moment on, her eyes never left mine, and as I sang she mouthed the words along with me. The excitement in her eyes as we sang this classic melody was touching.

After we talked a bit more, she said she needed to rest. She did not want me to go, but she was feeling weak. Before I left, she said, "This is so wonderful. Thank you so much. You will never know how much this meant to me."

A RHYTHMIC CONVERSATION

A Patient with Autism

The client had a primary diagnosis of autism and was also blind and deaf. Understandably, interaction during sessions was difficult for this man. In my first one-on-one with him, the client entered the room and sat down. I sat in front of him and began playing the guitar so he could feel the vibrations. Once we made initial contact, he took my hands because he uses the presence of rings to identify individuals. I then began to play the guitar again, and he grabbed the instrument to feel the vibrations. I continued to play as he kept his hands on it, sometimes dampening the strings so that no pitches were played and it was just the vibration of the rhythmic strum.

When the client released the guitar, I placed jingle bells and an egg shaker on a table in front of him; he explored each instrument before making his selection. He chose the egg shaker, which he played close to his ear at a steady pace. I entrained with his rhythm, patting his leg as he played. He placed the egg shaker in a container on his table to indicate he was finished.

Next, I played steady quarter notes on a djembe. The client turned toward the vibration, and I placed his hands on the head of the drum so that he could feel its source. He timidly rubbed the head of the instrument, and I imitated his playing. Then I hit the drum once to see what kind of reaction I would get. He pulled back his hands, but then placed them on the drum and hit it twice. I imitated him and we continued in this fashion; we had a musical conversation. After each time he played, the client would remove his hands from the drum and rub his head.

This behavior has been observed and is assessed as his way of giving himself deep pressure stimulation. Our conversation continued for few minutes until he got restless and tried to get up from the chair.

The session lasted for ten minutes, longer than his usual patience and attention span. I decided it was time to stop, so I played and sang a goodbye song to him. He felt the vibrations by holding the guitar. For me, this monumental session demonstrated how music could reach someone who has no clear way of communicating. For a short time, we conversed using a musical language of vibrations.

DON'T JUDGE THE SURFACE
Interacting with a Man Who is Non-Verbal

A non-verbal patient was lying in bed, listening to our singing and moving his left arm back and forth. He reached out his arm toward me as if to shake my hand after the song ended, but his hand was held tightly in a fist. I touched his hand and said I was glad to meet him. I asked if he wanted another song; he immediately blinked both eyes.

While I wasn't sure if this was his way of communicating, it felt like a "Yes." We did two more songs, closing with "Somewhere Over the Rainbow." During the song, the patient's movements subsided and he fell asleep. When the song was over, I quietly thanked him and left the room. Even though the patient never spoke, I felt like I had communicated with him.

I learned to always expect more out of a patient, not less. This positive, open-mined approach may lead to more unique and beneficial interventions.

THE MUSIC SAYS IT ALL
Spanish-Speaking Breast Cancer Patient

The first two times I passed this patient's room, she was curled up in bed, fast asleep. After visiting several patients, something told me to go back one last time to check on her. She was up and moving around, so I asked if I could visit.

As I began speaking to her daughter, I quickly realized that none of the three women in the room spoke English and I would have to dust off my Spanish-language skills. I explained who I was as best I could and hoped that the family understood. She happily agreed to a music therapy session. The patient sat on the edge of her bed and listened intently as I explained which Spanish songs I knew and that she could choose any of them to begin our session.

She and her family members selected four songs that morning. While singing "Besame Mucho," the patient began to cry. She smiled during the other songs and asked her family to be quiet as we sang.

When she chose "La Bamba," I took out instruments and encouraged the patient and her family to play along with the music. During this song, a nurse came in and sang with us, making the experience enjoyable for all involved. After each song, they applauded and commented that the music was "bonita," which means "pretty" in Spanish. The patient thanked me heartily for coming to her room that day and asked if I could come back to see her another day.

At the start of this session, I had no idea what was in store for me. Communicating with people who do not speak your native tongue is challenging. In this case, I did not have a chance to get nervous before entering the room, since I caught the eye of all three women as I approached the door with a guitar strapped to my back. Being welcomed into the room even before getting the chance to explain whom I was or why I was roaming the halls with my guitar was wonderful.

From my intervention, I learned that spoken language is not always needed to touch a patient. Although our minor language barrier kept verbal communication to a minimum, the music we shared that day is what truly connected the patient, her family, and me.

COMMUNICATIVE CUE
Adolescent on the Autism Spectrum

My client's primary goal is to increase appropriate participation. His objective is to demonstrate participation four times per session by playing an instrument, making choices, making eye contact with a therapist, engaging in appropriate peer interactions, or fulfilling a task. When prompted by a musical phrase, he can independently complete it. He often leaves the group during the session due to behavioral issues and/or overstimulation. Overall, we aim to increase his duration of participation throughout the entire session.

This week's session was chaotic. Most of the students exhibited more behavioral problems than usual. The teachers described the client's inappropriate behaviors as, "loud hands, loud feet, and loud voice." He presented these behaviors prior to the session, yet they subsided during the "Hello Song" and several verbal prompts from his teacher.

The next music experience was a blues songwriting intervention. I improvised a verse pertaining to every individual. We first sang what each person was working on for the week and then sang a suggestion of how to make that situation better.

The client created the following song in a twelve-bar blues format: "Oh, I get so excited, yes I do. Oh I get so excited, how about you? When I get excited...I need quiet hands and voice."

For the line "I need quiet hands and voice," I decreased the volume and modeled the movement with the exaggerated motion of bringing my hands quietly onto his desk and resting them there. He imitated this movement and instantly calmed, sat quietly at his desk, and made direct eye contact. I looked to his teacher and she said, "We tell him 'quiet hands' or 'quiet voice' all the time, but he's never followed through like that."

The client had several outbursts throughout the session and the teacher continued to try verbal prompting. When these cues did not work, I sang the last line from the song and modeled the movement for him. This method was successful 100% of the time; therefore, the teachers and I agreed that it would be beneficial to record the musical phrase onto an audio-recorded switch.

The teachers planned to use the switch as a reminder for how he could redirect his behavior. They tried hand-over-hand with him to get him to be in control of the switch. At the end of the day, the teachers expressed their appreciation and said that it worked all day long. They are learning the blues tune that the client wrote and plan to use it with him to provide more in-the-moment support.

What a great example of how music can be used as a communication tool. I feel that I made a difference not only for the client, but also was able to provide a model for the teachers to more effectively communicate with him.

CHAPTER 2: QUESTIONS FOR GROWTH

1. In a few excerpts, the clients had limited capacity for communication, often limited to only eye contact and restricted movement. What resources are available to music therapists for such cases?

2. What are some music therapy interventions that can be used with patients who have hearing/visual impairment? Which instruments best accompany the interventions?

3. Describe a music therapy session experience where language was a barrier. Were you able to overcome it, and if so, how?

4. What different approaches can music therapists take when working with clients who have first languages other than that of the music therapist?

5. How important is language and facial expression of music therapists? Of clients?

6. Name different strategies that music therapists can use to limit/change negative self-talk.

7. What are some emotions that music can aid in processing, and which interventions can be used for the processing of those emotions?

Chapter 3 - Leave Yourself at the Door

"The state of your life is nothing more than a reflection of your state of mind."

— Dr. Wayne W. Dyer

Tears of Joy
Hospitalized Middle-Age Woman

While I try to project warmth toward patients, I typically walk into a room with a degree of professional and emotional distance. I do this in hopes of remaining objective so that I can implement interventions that are best for the patient. However, this patient's comments indicated she was benefitting from music therapy, making it particularly difficult to maintain emotional distance.

From reading her chart, I learned that this patient was a Catholic, bilingual woman who endured a long hospital stay after a motor vehicle accident caused by a drunk driver. Even before meeting her, my heart went out to her, and I wondered if I could meet her needs and remain objective.

After knocking on the door, the patient appeared fatigued yet emanated joy. I offered music therapy services, which she accepted. She reported pain, anxiety, and nausea at zero when I checked in. If it hadn't been for the referral for support due to a long hospital stay, I would not have thought this patient needed our services. However, I felt that I was supposed to be there. I asked her if she would like to hear some songs and she enthusiastically agreed. She had a strong command of the English language, so I felt simple songs in English would be most accessible and potentially beneficial for her.

I wasn't prepared for what happened as I began to sing. The patient immediately began crying but continued to smile. She said, "Thank you for bringing this beautiful voice to me. I am not crying because I am in pain, I am crying because I am so happy." This was almost too much for me.

Because of this woman's openness of spirit, I found myself so overwhelmed with emotion that I had to self-administer deep breathing techniques to avoid crying. I continued with other mellow songs while the patient drifted in and out of sleep. At the end of the third selection, I began to collect my things. Music therapy seemed, at the very least, to have facilitated relaxation. She opened her eyes and said, "Thank you. I love what you've brought to me."

LET IT GO INTO THE DRUM
Clients with Eating Disorders/Substance Abuse

I had planned a session for active music making, but as my co-therapist and I were setting up, we overheard one of the guests speaking angrily with one of the workers. The atmosphere in the facility was heated. We discussed that we needed to be flexible to make this session work. We had planned to ask the clients if they had reflected on anything from last week's group, but scrapped it since their current moods and feelings appeared to be very present.

I stepped out of the room to check in with the staff. One client was sitting at a computer and I asked her how she was doing. She replied that she was having a bad day and she didn't feel up to music therapy. I told her that we wanted her to join, but she declined.

Another client came into the session. She said she felt "upset." We played "upset" on the drum together, then representations of each other's feelings, leading into a drumming improvisation. Following her lead, the drumming quickly got loud and fast. Within minutes, we were all screaming and beating on the drum.

Soon after we called "4-3-2-1 stop," the client who had declined to join the group opened the door and asked, "Are you guys going to continue to drum?" I told her we were, and she asked to join the session. She came in, grabbed a drum, and sat down. We played her feeling: "Empty."

We went into another drumming improvisation. Again, we screamed and beat the drums. Then, we played the marimbas and slit drums. For the last round, we asked the clients to play while thinking about a strength they hold within them.

Lessons Learned

"No matter how much preparation is put into the session plan, it will never work better than being present and flexible for the clients' needs."

For our check out, both girls spoke of overcoming difficult obstacles and being proud for not giving up.

I am regularly challenged to be flexible. I threw the session plan out the window and did what the group needed. The power of music constantly amazes me. It called to a client that initially declined and allowed her to express herself. The other client released anger and tension by drumming. Both said that they felt calm and relaxed after the session.

STEP ASIDE AND LET MUSIC
Client with Autism

My client seemed withdrawn from the group. During the greeting song, he reluctantly acknowledged me with eye contact and facial expression when prompted by his teacher. The second activity focused on active music making with the paddle drum, to which he exhibited little response.

Near the end of this activity, his teacher left the room. I was willing to try anything that would encourage him to reach his goal of engagement. I grabbed an ocean drum and slowly tilted it back and forth, creating a soothing sound. The client instantly looked up, holding his head in his hands, and watched closely as I facilitated the activity with another group member.

With his teacher still absent, I cautiously made my way over to him and presented him with the ocean drum. I moved it from side to side, and he reached out for it with his left hand and then quickly retracted it. I gave it a light tap with my right hand, as to mirror his left side, still offering the drum to him with my left hand.

He reached out again with his left hand and made contact with the rim. I stopped tapping my hand that still touched the drum rim - and waited. He tapped quickly three times and stopped. I tapped back, mimicking his exact pattern. The client then tapped a new pattern, which I mimicked.

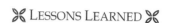

✂ LESSONS LEARNED ✂

"This encounter reinforced my belief that every diagnosed disability possesses many special abilities, unique to each client."

This went back and forth a few times, until he began improvising extended measures with both hands. I began providing supportive sound by slowly moving the ocean drum back and forth while he was playing it, encouraging him to hear both sounds and move with the drum.

At this point, the teacher came back in and was astounded at his involvement. I quietly asked her if it was too much stimulation, and she said, "No, please keep going!" We played until he was finished and indicated so by placing his hands over his head once again.

This "aha" moment for me demonstrated the magic and power of the musical relationship between client and therapist. I am there to facilitate music and lead activities, but allowing him to take the lead and guide me in a call and response provided him control over his environment and a sense of mastery.

STEP OUT OF YOUR SHELL

A Young Girl – Part of State Services

I was leading a group of children involved in the Department of Social Services Family Assisted Services system. For several weeks, the group worked on a songwriting project on the topic of the problems of the world and what we can do to make it better, appropriately named, "Dreamin' of a Better Place."

Four group members consistently attend, but this week, a shy and reserved adolescent girl was the only one present. The session focused on the recording element of the songwriting process. The girl rarely sang in front of the other group members, so this session was a great opportunity to get her out of her shell by singing and recording her voice.

As the session began, the client presented with a shy disposition; she spoke quietly and avoided eye contact. We drummed along to our composed beat as it played through the speakers. I asked her if we could rap her verse together over the beat while we were playing. She nodded and we began rapping, but she was very quiet. I lowered my voice to encourage her to add volume. At first, she remained quiet, and then she began to steadily increase her volume until ours matched.

We repeated her verse three times, and then I added the hook, "Dreamin' of a better place... dreamin' of a better place." Her verse ended, but I kept singing. I nodded and smiled at the client, and she began to sing. This was the first time I had heard her singing voice over the past month, and it was wonderful.

After a few times singing through the hook, she said she felt ready to record if I rapped and sung it with her. I agreed, but told her that I wanted her to be a bit louder than me since it was her words we were singing. She agreed.

We laid down the track in three takes and the client expressed that it was "cool" to record and then hear it play back. "That's what I sound like?" she asked. I said, "Yeah, pretty professional, huh?" She smiled and nodded. She asked for a CD to take home for her mom because they had discussed what we were doing and her mother was excited to hear what she had created. The client was proud to bring this finished product home to her mother and grateful for the opportunity to have some personal music time.

I learned that as a music therapist, I should not let low attendance at group sessions discourage me, but instead embrace the member in attendance and make the most of the more intimate setting. Everything happens for a reason. That girl was meant to be alone in this session so she would have the opportunity for individual recording and let her voice be heard.

MAGIC OF THE MOMENT
An Elderly Woman with Physical Ailments

I watched the patient slowly roll down the hallway in her wheelchair, pushing her walker and running out of breath; I wondered whether I would have time to see her before I left. And after two sessions with other patients, my co-therapist and I had time to stop in to see her.

We asked the patient if she wanted to participate in a music-centered relaxation exercise, she responded with a faint and weary "yes." She presented with shortness of breath and looked uncomfortable as her hands shook below her tense shoulders. She called out desperately to the nurse for more meds before we began the exercise. I encouraged her to physically readjust to find a more comfortable position and close her eyes.

My co-therapist and I sang rhythmic phrases: "breathe in" (major chord), "hold" (musical tension), "breathe out" (musical resolve to tonic). Soon, the patient matched her breath to follow the music we provided. The cycle seemed so natural, especially the dissonant sonority paired with the patient's exhale. I kept a close watch on the patient as we continued the cycle, and her furrowed brow relaxed. Less sweat glistening on her face and her breath slowed and deepened within her chest.

When we stopped, she opened her eyes and said with a smile, "I didn't know music could do that. That was great." She had never heard of music therapy. We then moved on to toning and continued relaxation exercises. A couple of days later, she was happy to see us when we returned to do more relaxation exercises with her.

Keeping the patient as the center is so important in therapy. This seems like common sense, but remembering that (ideally) every occurrence during a session happens in the present for the patient is hard. I realized that at the same time this experience was exciting for me as the therapist, it was everything for the client. All of my concerns of the day were unimportant when we were in the moment.

GO WITH THE FLOW

An Inconsolable Woman Referred for Agitation

A patient was referred to us for agitation. When my co-therapist and I arrived, she was sitting in a chair. Before we had an opportunity to greet her, she expressed a desire to stand, thereby setting off alarms on one of her machines. I encouraged her to sit while waiting for the medical staff to investigate the cause of the alarm, as I was unaware if the patient was allowed to get out of the chair. Her nurse entered the room to check the machines and requested that the patient sit. The patient responded, "I'll sit down when I'm ready to sit down."

Immediately, another member of the medical staff came in and asked her to sit down, to which the patient again indicated her preference to stand. The staff asked my co-therapist to stand near the patient to help steady her, if need be. I introduced myself and invited the patient to identify her preferred music, to which the patient responded that she could not hear me. I moved closer, speaking louder, and repeated the invitation. The patient stated that she did not know of any songs and refused the invitation to choose from a list of selected songs, as she did not have her glasses.

I began to play "Edelweiss." After several measures, I asked the patient if she recognized the song; she did not. After noticing her looking at the kalimba, my co-therapist invited her to try playing it. The patient refused the invitation, asking the therapists to play a song for her instead. My co-therapists and I improvised a piece on guitar and kalimba for a few minutes. During this piece, another member of the medical staff entered the patient's room and invited her to sit, to which she replied, "Thank you for the thirty-third invitation, but I will sit when I'm ready." My co-therapist was once again instructed to keep an eye on the patient as she stood.

We continued our improvisation and during the music, the patient chose to sit. Once the song ended, I asked her if she played any instruments. She replied, "All good American girls play an instrument - the piano." Further attempts to engage her in conversation regarding her musical background were met with such responses as, "If I wanted to hear a lecture on music, I would ask for one, but what's the point? Do you have another song?" My co-therapist and I decided to play "Five Foot Two" in an attempt to elicit a relaxed and positive response from the patient. She began speaking during the song, so I stopped the accompaniment to understand what she was saying. The patient indicated that she wished for the session to end by saying, "This has been nice, but I don't think we will explore this any further."

I felt frustrated because I wanted to give the patient what I assessed that she needed, but I couldn't figure out how to do so. We tried to follow her lead based on comments she made and her responses, but it seemed that nothing we were doing pleased her. As therapists, our flexibility during the session was so important. I learned that awareness of what I'm experiencing should be noted, but then let go of, so that my feelings don't affect the session.

HOLD MY HAND

A Woman Suffering from a Foot Abscess Due to Diabetes

When I entered the room, the patient was thoroughly excited. She said, "I thought no one would be able to come by and see me until tomorrow. I am so glad that you are here."

I asked the patient what her pain level was on a scale of 1-10 (1 = no pain, 10 = severe pain). She rated her pain at a 5, which she said was "pretty bad". She then picked some of her favorite songs from my book, and we sang them together. Between each song, we talked of her memories of home, family, work, and hobbies. This delightful woman had many lessons and stories to share. She spoke of her illness, describing the spasms and shooting pain.

After a few more songs, she looked at me and told me that she felt one of her spasms coming on. She told me not to worry if she began to cry, because it always happened when her spasms occurred. Within seconds, her entire body began to cringe in pain. She reached her hand out to me, and I wrapped both of my hands around hers. I then began to sing soft, improvisatory music to her. She stayed focused on me and continued to breathe while pain shot through her body. I kept singing.

When the pains ceased after a few minutes, I maintained the grip on her hand. She looked at me and said, "That is the first time I haven't cried." I was so moved. She continued, "When you sing, it helps my pain go away."

We closed the session by singing a few more songs of her choice. I asked the patient where her pain level was again, this time she replied that it was at a 1 out of 10. As we wrapped up our time together, she reached her hand out to mine once again. I told her that it was a pleasure to spend part of my day with her, and she said the same. "You know, I prayed today for a special blessing, and I know that you were sent to me."

One can never know how powerful of an impact music therapy can have on the patients. The session was a reminder to always be in the moment and do everything possible to 'be there' for the patient.

FREEDOM THROUGH MUSIC
Inmate with a Ruptured Spleen

A nurse who often gave me referrals asked me to see a patient of hers. "He's going to turn you down," she warned. She asked if I would go in anyway and play for him, stating that he really needed it and she would come in with me.

On our way to his room, the nurse informed me that the patient was a prison inmate and had been beaten up. She entered the room while I pulled out my guitar from the case, and I heard him yelling and moaning. She asked him if he would he let me come in for just one song. He yelled, "No! I don't want it. I just don't want to be in pain anymore!"

I stood in the doorway, unsure about what to do. He was hand-cuffed to the bed and a prison guard stood in the corner of his room. The nurse tried to convince him to let me enter several times, and finally he conceded, "OK, just one song."

I walked over to his bedside and introduced myself. His breathing was quick and labored. I told him I would try to help with the pain, and I attempted a relaxation exercise. I told him to listen to the music and take deep breaths while trying to pace his breathing with the music. He got a little quieter and his breathing slowed, although he still winced in pain and groaned now and then. He watched me play, and at one point said, "That's a D ... a G," recognizing the chords I was playing. I remarked that he must be a guitarist.

> **LESSONS LEARNED**
>
> *"Music allows people to step outside of the hospital environment into a place of comfort and familiarity. It allows a sense of control in a place where everyone else is making decisions for you."*

Eventually, his groaning lessened and in short, occasional sentences, he told me about the guitars he owned and the music he liked. He requested a song, and I began to play. He said he played it differently and asked if he could play the guitar. I placed the guitar in his lap and he played for about five minutes. When he was done, he thanked me and said he really enjoyed it. He agreed to a final song. With his approval, I sang "Three Little Birds." He nodded his head and joined me in a quiet, gentle voice, "Every little thing's going to be all right – they're going to take out my spleen..."

It was an emotional moment and I felt tears behind my eyes. I turned around to leave and was faced with a group of nurses and other staff members gathered around the doorway. They congratulated the patient on his playing and applauded. The nurses were amazed at his behavior, saying that was the first time they had ever seen him smile. I was then told that he was one of the most difficult patients they'd ever had – very uncooperative and resistant to anything they tried to do. "You have no idea how good this was for him," a nurse said.

I felt a sense of humility that day and privileged that this patient, in particular, allowed me into his world – an interaction that was only able to occur through the music. Music bridges a gap between people and allows a relationship to form that would not otherwise be possible.

GENERATION GAP
Female in Short-Term Care

My patient was an 82-year-old woman who came into the hospital for a short-term treatment. We did three songs of her choice, with small "ice-breaker" comments and verbal interactions in between. She told me to play something of my own choice – something that I liked. I decided to play my favorite song from when I was a teenager.

When I finished playing, I saw she had enjoyed the song. "That was beautiful!" she said. She also stated that she was going to look for music by that band. She began to talk about the song, saying it was an appropriate and comforting song for anybody in a hospital. I agreed and added that it was an appropriate song for anyone going through difficult times or loneliness.

She said she was experiencing a lot of loneliness after her husband's death earlier in the year. With this, she broke into tears. She talked about how she missed him, how her life had this huge void, about their long and wonderful marriage, their children, and how hard it was to be without him. My reaction at the moment was to stay there and be receptive to her expression during this deep and emotional experience. I appreciate the fact that she opened up to me in this way.

Afterward, I felt my typical tendency to judge myself and question whether I had acted appropriately. I wondered if I should have said or done something different. The moment was perfect as it was, just because it was what was felt. I sometimes console or try to alleviate someone's emotional pain because I feel uncomfortable with the open expression of suffering. I think it was a good thing to just step back and allow for her to take all the space she needed to express her feelings, while still acknowledging the moment.

I am reminded of something that I once heard someone say: "The best gift that we can give to another is the quality of our attention."

DARKNESS TO LIGHT
Woman with a Small Bowel Obstruction

The first time I checked the room, the patient was not there. When I went back, I entered and noticed the woman's confused demeanor. I introduced myself and asked if she was in any pain or had any anxiety. She stated that she had neither pain nor anxiety, but she was tired because of her recent shower. I suggested music for relaxation and I began facilitating a relaxation exercise while improvising on the guitar.

The patient stopped me after about five minutes to tell me that she was more relaxed and that she would love to hear one of the songs we were playing earlier for her neighbor. I named the two songs we had sung for the other patient, and she chose "I Can't Help Falling in Love with You." As I sang, I noticed that she had begun to cry. The crying turned into sobbing, so I retrieved a tissue and sat holding her hand, continuing to sing. She began to tell me how much she missed her husband who died two years earlier. The last time she was in the hospital, he was with her. He became sick shortly after that. She continued to cry, and we sat in the moment together.

> ✂ LESSONS LEARNED ✂
>
> *"It is often more important to be in the moment with the client than to continue with the session in a paced way."*

After she finished sharing her memories and was ready to move out of the sadness, I asked if she wanted me to continue singing the song, which she did. When I finished, she thanked me and chose more upbeat songs, including "YMCA." She even moved her arms to the song along with me.

I have learned to be more humanistic through my internship. The doctors, nurses, physical therapists, and social workers seem to often rush around, trying to accomplish tasks on their agendas. Music therapists can be there for the client or patient in whichever way they want or need us, even if that means sitting in the moment and being present to the sadness with them. I could sit with her and lift her mood once she was ready.

FEELING THE LOVE
Retired Pastor with Coronary Disease

I accepted the opportunity to see a patient per my supervisor's request. He is a retired pastor who has experienced recent coronary disease. My hymn repertoire was rather small, so I decided to practice a few hymns before going to the session, not knowing whether we would even use them. When I arrived, his family spotted me and asked, "Is that a guitar?" They didn't know that the patient had requested music and were happy that the guitar was coming into their room.

The patient was weak and could only speak softly, but he could still communicate his likes and dislikes. Everyone in the room was musical - his wife and daughter both sang beautifully and harmonized from time to time. Everyone joined in to sing one song, including the patient, and suddenly I felt as though someone was behind me. Thinking it was the medical staff, I looked back, but no one was there. I relaxed again. Seconds later, I experienced the same feeling. It happened a few more times, but every time I looked back, no one was there. The two women talked to me afterward, saying that a smiling spirit was in the room. The women saw me reacting and knew what was happening. I'm not sure what I think it was, but it was definitely interesting.

We took time to write an original short song. I suggested a prayer or something similar. Collectively, the family decided on "Be still and know that I am God." The eight slow measures sounded beautiful. We surrounded the patient's bed and all repeated the song several times.

I departed with hugs and kisses from the family. The patient blew me a kiss and asked his daughter to kiss me for him. What a loving, supportive, and spiritual environment. My co-therapist returned to the critical care unit the following day to follow up with the patient. Upon arriving, the patient's wife told him the following story:

"When the music therapist left here yesterday, his [the patient's] condition improved suddenly and has remained improved since. Not only that, but other patients in the CCU heard the music and it positively affected them as well. The nurse had told me that yesterday morning had been stressful, but the music seemed to relax everyone in the unit, patients and nurses alike! Thank her again for us."

THE TOOLBELT
Male with Esophageal Perforation

I had been seeing a referred patient for almost a month. My initial visit was designed as a diversion from his long stay in the hospital environment since he did not report pain or anxiety. However, during different sessions, the patient started expressing feelings and concerns he was beginning to identify and acknowledge.

Each week, the patient mentioned how he used to play the piano, to which I finally responded, "Why don't I bring the keyboard here so you can play?" The day I brought the keyboard, he was lying in bed and did not want to move, so I changed my plans. In previous sessions, we had discussed writing a song about the chicken bone that caused the perforation in his esophagus. This day, he responded that he was not in the mood to write a song, which was unusual for him.

"OK, so my backup plan isn't working," I thought. As I assessed the situation, the patient's visitor kept insisting on something "happy." I did not know why she was so insistent on this type of music until I found out the patient was having surgery later that day.

I selected "I Can See Clearly Now" to satisfy the visitor's request, but also knowing that the patient may not be in a "happy" mood, I prepared to do some songwriting. During the process, we used positive affirmations and other songwriting tools. The patient responded by singing, "It is a bright, bright sun shining day." He added some of his own words in the song, and tears began to form in his eyes.

This patient clearly had a lot of anxiety about his upcoming surgery, which explained his lack of enthusiasm. Thinking in the moment and being flexible allowed me to throw out my initial plans and meet the patient where he was in the present. This attitude paved the way for a session that benefitted the patient by providing what he needed. Sometimes plans do not go accordingly, but sessions can still be successful with in-the-moment adaptations. If I think back to the first sessions I led in practicum, I probably would have frozen up when faced with improvising a session. It reassures me that all of my education and internship experiences have prepared me for the unexpected, and I am truly developing a music therapy tool belt of skills that I can use in any situation.

CHAPTER 3: QUESTIONS FOR GROWTH

1. As a music therapist, what is the importance of maintaining emotional distance in sessions?

2. In one of the excerpts from this chapter, a group session was planned for, yet only one individual showed up. How can you adapt planned group experiences such as a drum circle for just one client? Get into small groups and roleplay with your peers. Present different scenarios where a session plan is no longer an option. At the end, discuss the outcomes among the group.

3. How can you be present for clients in a large group with varying needs? Does the obvious need of one client outweigh the needs of all the rest enough for the therapist to be present rather than objective?

4. Look up the concept of humanism and take a moment to reflect on a past session in which the client had an emotional reaction. In what ways can you make your clinical interactions more humanistic?

5. A few different terms and diagnoses have been used in this chapter. Define the following:
    a. Uterine cancer,
    b. Acute renal failure,
    c. Rheumatoid arthritis,
    d. William's syndrome,
    e. Small bowel obstruction,

f.   Coronary disease, and

g.   Esophageal perforation.

6. In "Go With The Flow," is there anything that could have been done differently by the therapy team to facilitate another outcome?

CHAPTER 4 - FORGET ABOUT IT

"You have first to experience what you want to express."

—Vincent van G

BLIND SESSION
Male with Mystery Diagnosis

As I walked through the halls of the oncology unit looking for a previous patient's room, I heard someone say, "Hey! You should come in here!" I peeked in the room, and the nurse asked me if I was still seeing people. I stated that I was and the middle-aged man in the bed gave me a smile. He appeared alert and looked stable and healthy.

I set up and asked him if there were any songs that he would like to hear. He requested "Bridge Over Troubled Water." The song is somewhat depressing, yet comforting, so I thought I understood why he chose it. We never discussed his diagnosis, which was most likely cancer due to his placement in oncology. He was pleasant and funny, and throughout the session, I was curious about why he was there.

After one song, he didn't want any more music, so I thanked him, his wife, and the nurse who had been listening. I noticed that the energy in the room wasn't negative. When I looked at his chart I learned that he was in the hospital for mental instability. Earlier in his life, he had been kidnapped for 30 hours, and he developed post-traumatic stress disorder (PTSD) and he has a tremor.

He claimed to be blind in one eye, but the doctors couldn't find anything physiologically wrong with his vision. His fingers and toes lock up in strange positions for hours at a time.

I learned that I really can never know what a person is in the hospital for before seeing their chart. This man's chart revealed much more about him than I could glean from just walking into the room. Going into a session blind was an interesting experience for me.

DIFFERENCES APART
Uterine Cancer Patient

I had visited all of the patients on my list for the day and was preparing to leave when I ran into a nurse. She asked me if I had seen a particular patient, which I hadn't because her cancer diagnosis was not listed on the census.

The nurse informed me that this patient did not have health insurance and that the county and state were funding her hospital stay and procedures. The nurse explained that the patient most likely would not be here the next week because state funding agencies tend to cycle patients through the system quickly. The nurse also told me that the patient was interested in music therapy and practiced a lot of alternative therapies.

Based on my previous contact with people who are involved in holistic and alternative therapies, I had a stereotype in mind of what this patient might be like. Immediately upon entering her room, and even before I could get one word out, she saw me with my guitar and said, "Sit down and play me something!" as she cleared a spot for me at the foot of her bed. I pulled up a chair next to the bed. We talked for nearly the entire session. She told me about herself, her life, and other concerns she was having.

We only made music twice. First, we made up our own lyrics to the blues, and then sang one song together. Throughout our session, the patient briefly spoke with one or two people on the phone and a couple of medical staff who came in her room to check on her.

During the course of my visit with her, I realized that she was one of the kindest, most genuine, and sincerest people I have ever met. She spoke with love, warmth, and kindness on the phone, to medical staff, and to me.

I came into this session expecting to talk about concepts regarding holistic health and alternative therapies. I learned that preconceived ideas about a patient don't accomplish anything and isn't a catalyst for anything good... it is actually a hindrance.

A SPECIAL VISIT
Woman with Acute Renal Failure

My experience with this patient happened almost by accident, when her son spotted one of the music therapists outside of a room tuning a guitar. "You've got to go see my mother," he said. "She loves music."

The patient shared with us her love for classical music and her despair of being in the hospital. My co-therapist and I began the session with a few songs that the patient chose, for which she and her husband were quite thankful. When I told her I had brought along my cello, her face brightened and her eyes swelled with tears of happiness. "I love the violin," she told us. "Would you play something for me?" I told her I would be delighted and I started to set up.

The moment I began to play a slow, lyrical improvisation, the patient burst into tears, overflowing with emotion. She assured me that she was fine. She hadn't heard the cello in a long time and the sound of it - just for her - in her hospital room was overwhelming. "This is a miracle," she said. "I never expected in my wildest imagination that I would hear this in my hospital room!" I continued to play for several minutes, allowing her to release the tears that I assumed had been building up inside her.

I asked her about her love of the violin and she told me that years ago, her nephew used to practice his violin in her garden at home. She had enjoyed his private concerts immensely and the sound of the instrument brought back those moments. Her tears were those of joy. Before we left, she said, "You are both angels. Thank you so much for coming, and please come see me again." Never before had my cello playing brought someone to tears or been so appreciated.

THE PRIMARY INSTRUMENT
Classroom with Developmental Disabilities

I had a placement at a center for children and adults with developmental disabilities. I decided to try something new, something maybe the students had never seen or experienced. Therapists often need different interventions to grab and maintain their attention.

I began all of my sessions by bringing out a large, black bag and asking, "Who knows what this is?" The group studied it carefully, yelling out answers like, "Guitar!" or "Violin!" or "Drum!" This session, I slowly uncovered the hidden object, revealing the reddish-gold wood underneath. They watched quite intently as the new object appeared; many of them seemed to know what it was, but could not pinpoint the name. I gave them various hints, trying to trigger their memories.

Finally, it was time to reveal the name. "This is a cello," I carefully pronounced. I gave them a basic introduction to the instrument, explaining how the sound is produced and the different ways to make it. I also used the opportunity for the students to practice recognizing differences in two similar objects by holding up the guitar and asking which one had more strings and which one was bigger.

The bow was an interesting object to them as well, and when I asked what they thought it was, I got some close answers like, "A stick." When I asked what they thought the white, smooth part of the bow was, someone said, "Hair!"

We proceeded to play several listening games, like "Name That Tune," and a new game where they raised and lowered their hands based upon the high or low notes I was playing; however, the most interesting game involved the students taking turns conducting me. When I asked who would like to try, one student leaned forward and shot up his hand.

With little instruction, he stood up and raised his arms. And with a look of anticipation in his eyes, he began to move his hands above his head, very quickly. I responded with high, staccato notes. At this, his face lit up and a smile spread across his face. He continued to conduct, quite accurately and with very deliberate cues for different musical dynamics including loud, soft, fast, and slow. He then stopped me and sat down. His face was beaming with pride as he looked at his teacher for approval and everyone clapped.

This response was amazing to me as this particular student rarely smiled and often looked at me with a blank stare. This was the first time I had ever seen him smile so brightly in all the months I had been working with him. "The cello works!" I thought.

The power of my principal instrument never ceases to amaze me. The cello seems to reach everyone - old and young, healthy and sick. Its therapeutic properties are apparent in its human-like shape and sound and its accessibility for all to play, even if it's just a pull of a string.

WHAT WORKS FOR THE PATIENT, WORKS FOR YOU
An Open-Minded Patient and Therapist

This woman was by far the most accepting and open patient that I have treated in the hospital. In this specific session, I wanted to address her physical symptoms because our initial session together focused on emotional release.

I brought Tibetan and crystal toning bowls and as the session began, she told me that she had just finished her in-bed yoga workout and she was ready for relaxation. I learned that the client was a massage therapist, and we discussed holistic medicine for about ten minutes. I noticed how happy she appeared, almost like a different person from the last time I had seen her. She glowed and displayed positive affect. She told me that a few hours after our first session, her chest tube began flowing with fluids and almost filled her container. She reported how amazing this seemed to her because her body had not been kicking out a lot of fluids prior to our visit.

For this session, we began with a relaxation exercise involving deep breathing. As the exercise ended, she said she was so relaxed she almost fell asleep. She explained that she was so focused she felt like she was out of the hospital, and she also forgot about her chest tube bubbling in the background. We then moved into a lesson in toning, sending vibrations to break up unwanted tension or blockages in different areas of the body.

I don't like toning, but other people sometimes do. I never imagined that I would take toning bowls into the hospital and actually lead a session. But nonetheless, I knew from her symptoms that it was a good idea and a great way for her to work on breathing and releasing her blocked energy and stress. I always promote deep breathing and singing as therapy, and this day I was able to see those efforts come to fruition as the client benefitted and had so much fun — as did I.

POWER OF AN INSTRUMENT
A Withdrawn Male with Autism

My supervisor had asked me to prepare a session using my flute for my higher functioning group at a center for children and adults with profound developmental disabilities. I was a little skeptical because I had never used my flute before to lead every session activity. I was also concerned because playing my flute takes away my voice.

I designed a session plan in which I would conduct a very short lesson about the flute: where it is from, how old it is, what it was first made of, and where it is played. I had the students tell me whether I was playing up or down so that they would have to use their ears and not their eyes.

I was so impressed by one particular client. He usually keeps his eyes closed and has to sit by the teacher. He would play instruments if given the opportunity, but he made minimal eye contact and rarely spoke. I had asked his teacher the previous week to not sit next to the client for the session because I was curious how this would affect his participation. To my surprise, the minute I pulled out my flute the client opened his eyes and was completely focused.

Each opportunity I gave him to listen to the flute and tell me if I was playing up or down, he was correct. I also played a small number of notes on the flute and asked the clients how many I played.

This intervention was difficult for most clients, but this particular young man answered every question correctly. During a "Name That Tune" exercise, he identified "I've Been Working on the Railroad" and sang the entire song along with me while I played along. I was so amazed at the difference in his participation. I wish that I knew if his participation was attributed to the flute, the fact that he wasn't next to his teacher, or if it was just coincidence.

I discovered that the flute could work for more than relaxation. I had never thought about using my flute for educational purposes, let alone an entire music therapy session. Then I thought, "I can do this. It's just the flute and I know the flute."

It is interesting how the use of my principal instrument, which I never would have used with this population, would be the stimulus needed to reach that client.

CONFIDENCE

Working with an Unfamiliar Population

I worked with an adult diagnosed with developmental delay as well as deafness and blindness. I had seen her twice before, but this was my first interaction with her. I was intimidated because she was frantic and seemed aggressive. She obviously wanted her own space, hitting the table with her hands and feeling around her to make sure she was alone most of the time.

My supervisor showed me that the way to interact with this client is to approach her from behind, gently touch her arms and use the ASL signs for music, more, and good work. The sole music therapy goal for this client is to increase participation by instructing her to hit a paddle drum with a mallet.

It was my turn to initiate music therapy with the client. I was not excited about this because I was afraid to approach her. It took me a minute to compose myself, and then I jumped right in.

Immediately, I tensed and forgot what the signs were because I was too concerned with protecting myself. I was not ready to get hit in the face. I figured it out, but worried that if I wasn't doing the signs correctly or if I was taking too much time, the client would get frustrated and become aggressive. She did hit the drum four times with my cueing.

Before internship, I had never worked with clients who had developmental disabilities. Working with an individual who is both deaf and blind with additional diagnoses was a huge revelation for me.

I learned that I should not be intimidated and should jump right in when working with this client and other clients with compounded disabilities. I will be working with her every week one-on-one and need to be able to push aside my preconceived ideas.

SURPRISE
Child with William's Syndrome

I was growing frustrated with my case study. I had been working with this client for more than eight weeks, but I felt as though I couldn't see much progress during music therapy sessions.

Over the last few sessions, her attention to task was very short and I had difficulty getting her to complete one short intervention. One of her goals was learning to identify colors and the other was counting to ten. I had realized during a previous session that she seemed to be able to receptively identify her colors, but she could not expressively identify them. For example, when I asked her to put the blue beanbag on the blue drum or to point to the brown bear, she was able to do it correctly. However, she was not able to tell me the color of a scarf or other object when asked, "Which color do you want?"

Her progress on her counting goal was similar. I had heard her count from one to three by rote, but after that she was unable to count any higher with the numbers in the correct order. I had made a CD for her with some counting songs on it, and she seemed to enjoy one in particular, called "Jump and Count."

This week, I started the tape trying to find a different song, and when I hit play, it was in the middle of the counting song. It only played for a few seconds, but it started right at the counting section. The client heard the recording, "When we count to 8! 1, 2, 3, 4...." I turned it off after 4, but the client continued to count on her own, up to 8, in the right order. I had never heard her do this before, so I immediately reinforced the counting and asked her if she would like to sing that song instead of the other song I had been trying to find. She said, "Yes," and we started the tape again and began singing. She was able to sing the entire song, with all of the counting sections in the correct order. I was amazed.

After that song, we transitioned to a movement intervention using scarves. I held up two scarves in front of her and said, "Which color do you want?" To my amazement, she said, "Yellow," and reached up to take the yellow scarf. This was the first time I had ever seen her expressively identify a color. When I told her mother this later, she said excitedly that she didn't think she had ever heard her daughter say the word "Yellow."

Sometimes it takes a while to see observable results of music therapy with a client. When working with children with special needs, remember not to overlook what first may appear to be the smallest of accomplishments, because for these children it may be the first step toward a larger milestone. It is important to be patient and not grow frustrated or feel as though it is not effective.

IT'S JUST YOU AND THE CLIENT
Hospitalized Woman with Gastrointestinal Problems

I went to see an elderly woman referred by her nurse because she had been in a lot of pain over the past week. She was diagnosed with multiple ailments including a severe gastrointestinal infection and rheumatoid arthritis. Her nurse found me as soon as I stepped foot onto the hospital floor. She told me that they were having a difficult time with the patient and that she was in so much pain... no medication seemed to bring her enough comfort to calm her or provide relief. She said that this patient was very resistant to many of the nurses and physicians and that she would most likely decline music therapy services.

I put on my gown and gloves, thinking, "I'm just going to take these off in a second when she declines." I wondered whether this was a waste of time to even try with this patient because her nurse had set up the situation as if she was sure that my attempt would fail. I stopped and thought, "What am I doing? Why am I thinking this way? I should never judge a patient in any way before I go in the room."

I entered the room as if the nurse had not given me any information about the patient. We ended up having an amazing session during which the patient was able to relax for the first time in days. She ended up having fun and she said the session was "Extremely surprising and satisfying." She said she hadn't smiled in days until I came in and brightened her day.

I must never let anyone or anything create any preconceived notions or judgments about patients. As in this case, I shouldn't have let the nurse's comments about her patient affect the way I approached the room, the patient, or the session.

CHAPTER 4: QUESTIONS FOR GROWTH

1. In "Differences Apart," the author writes about holistic and alternative therapies. List a few alternative therapies.

2. What unconventional instruments can be used for music therapy and how? For example: in this chapter, some music therapists were able to utilize their principal instruments, the cello and the flute. Considering your principal instrument, what are some ways that you can plan an entire session around it? If your principal instrument is guitar, piano, or voice, what are unique ways you can use those instruments or other unconventional instruments and how?

3. How can music lessons serve as music therapy? How can music therapists make them clinical?

4. Working with unfamiliar populations is bound to happen. Thinking of the most unfamiliar population to you right now, what are some ways in which you can prepare for working with this population?

5. What are some preconceived ideas about your preferred population? How have preconceived ideas kept you from facilitating a certain experience or choosing a certain song?

Chapter 5 · The Elevator Pitch

> *"Now we're in the midst of not just advocating for change, not just calling for change — we're doing the grinding, sometimes frustrating work of delivering change.*
> *Inch by inch, day by day."*
>
> —*Former President Barack Obama*

The Proof is in the Pudding

Unresponsive Patient with Lymphoma

Newton's Third Law states that for each and every action there is an equal and opposite reaction. I don't think much about that; I take it for granted most days. When I do pause and ponder it, most events that come to mind are in the physical realm.

An experience I had with a patient sparked a light bulb moment for me: much of Newton's Third Law must be taken by faith. That is, we must believe that the effects of our efforts as music therapists are real, despite a lack of immediate physical or behavioral evidence.

The patient was sleeping in her bed. She was in isolation, did not socialize much, and her door was always closed; therefore, the typical hospital noises and nurses' voices were nearly silenced.

I decided to take a chance and invest some time with this patient, despite the fact that my research-oriented mind naturally seeks feedback. I softly sang and played guitar for about thirty minutes, keeping my eyes mostly locked onto the patient, searching for signs of response. There were none.

So, what was the outcome? What do I put down in the medical chart? What do I document? How do I justify my time with this patient? I don't. I can't. I follow my heart and my intuition, and I trust that the patient received some comfort, some distraction, and some reassurance that someone cared enough to spend time with her.

If Newton was right, the patient received every microgram of love and caring energy that I sent her way.

A SILENT OBSERVER
Patient Diagnosed with Breast Cancer

As I was finishing some charts, I hurried down the hallway to meet with my co-therapist who was a few minutes into an intervention. As I approached the patient's room, I heard her begin the first song.

Not wanting to barge in and distract or confuse the patient, I waited outside. As I sat and admired my co-therapist's performance of "Joy to the World," I tried to put myself in the mindset of a non-music therapist. What do doctors, nurses, or other professionals think as they are walking past a room when the patient is receiving music therapy?

All at once, I could see two sides to music therapy. From the perspective of someone who understands the profession, the music therapist was offering an energizing dose of joy and hope to the patient. "Joy to the world...all the boys and girls...joy to the fishes in the deep blue sea ... joy to you and me."

Here in the midst of physical pain and emotional trauma, the music therapist was providing the patient with an opportunity to focus on feeling good and thinking positively. Peace of mind is hard to come by in the hospital setting; however, music therapy can to provide just that.

From the perspective of someone who does not understand what music therapy is, however, the whole thing could seem trivial. At best, music could be seen as a pleasant means for enhancing the overall ambiance of the hospital setting... not essential and possibly not even reimbursable. "Do they really go to school for four to six years to learn how to play requests? Couldn't we take the money that we are paying a music therapist and invest it into entertainment systems that would allow patients to hear their favorite songs and/or watch their favorite movies? What does listening to music have to do with cancer treatment, anyway?"

As I thought about both sides of the coin, I realized that music therapy - just like music itself - is not for everyone. Music therapy interventions in the oncology setting are dependent on amazingly complex interactions between thoughts, feelings, and physiological functioning.

Predicting, with any scientific certainty, how different patients might benefit from music therapy is impossible.

All we can do is try to offer the highest quality music and therapeutic experience possible.

DOUBTING YOURSELF
Adults in a Psychiatric Facility

As music therapists, we will struggle with certain things throughout our careers. For me, it is frustrating to feel as though the clients we work with are not affected by our services. Of course, they are affected in some way; however, if they do not physically or verbally respond, it is challenging to determine how they are achieving a non-musical goal through music.

A music therapist must be willing to accept that there will be sessions in which this happens. When a group or individual responds in a way that they never have before, it is clear that they benefited, then that will be a moment that will not be taken for granted. It reminds me why we are here and why we should not get discouraged.

A psychiatric facility can be an emotionally draining place to work. Patients will sometimes spend an entire session staring, as if they are looking right through the facilitator. It sometimes feels as if it was all for nothing, and it can be defeating to not observe a solid response.

I had an experience that helped it click in my head that I have to keep an optimistic attitude when working with this population. A lot of these individuals are internal processors; it is rare to feel as if the group has unified during a session. This is frustrating because there is little opportunity for individual attention. This population could benefit greatly from more one-on-one interactions because when the focus turns to one person, it is not long before the rest of the group loses its focus.

After my first visit, I jumped to the conclusion that I didn't like doing this work with this population. The atmosphere dragged me down emotionally and there was little evidence of a positive result coming from the sessions. My very last session was a group of mentally unstable individuals. The group started off with one patient insulting another, which caused them to retreat from the group in tears and anger. It feels defeating to have a group begin this way. How should I have handled it? How could I have helped both of these individuals stabilize their anger? Sometimes, however, these things work themselves out. The woman who left returned, and that in itself felt like a success.

During a drumming intervention, a woman began singing "Feelings." I began to play along with her on the piano while the rest of the group drummed along with us. Then, just about every group member began singing along with her whether or not they knew the song. The group was looking at each other and feeding off the energy in the room. It was the first time I felt true unity among a group and it had a powerful effect on my attitude.

❊ LESSONS LEARNED ❊

"Sometimes, we just have to trust and know that what we are doing is effective. It makes those feelings of self-doubt completely worth the moments of feeling successful."

We all want to make a difference; it is difficult to feel that difference if we cannot see it. Knowing the benefits and seeing the small things is what makes our profession so rewarding.

FACING THE CHALLENGE
Young Adults with Disabilities

Working with students who have developmental disabilities can be challenging. I conduct music therapy sessions with seven groups of students at a school; some of them are higher functioning, and some are severely disabled.

I realized that I spend more time planning for students with higher skills; I don't mean to discriminate against the ones who are more challenging. I tend to have a sense of reward and meaning of what I provide when I receive positive response from the recipients, including the depth of connection that I establish with them.

How much influence needs to be provided for students who are deaf and blind? I ask myself, "Does what I do mean anything to them?" The answer is "Yes!" Rationalizing what we do when students wander around in the classroom screaming or throwing instruments at the wall is tough. Yet, everything compensates when I see a smile on their faces or hear a happy squeal from them.

SOMETIMES YOU WIN, SOMETIMES YOU LOSE
Educating About Music Therapy

This was my second visit to this patient. He welcomed me, requested songs, and actively listened while I played the guitar. He told me that he used to play the trumpet in a band, and his father was a good trumpet player.

As I was talking to him, he asked me if we perform in services for weddings, receptions, and so forth... another misconception of music therapy. I explained to him what we do, how we are trained, and that music therapy is an established health care profession. Despite my attempt, I did not think that he fully understood what I did, although he seemed to appreciate my visit.

I visited another patient's room next. His girlfriend was leaving the room when I was going in. She said, "Oh music, he's going to enjoy that. Come on in."

The patient welcomed me and seemed excited about finding out about music therapy. He played the guitar and seemed interested in using music to cope with his disease. "I can't believe some people decline," the man said. He and his girlfriend asked me a lot of detailed questions, and I was happy to answer them.

During our conversation, the man remarked, "This is the best part of my day!" Afterward, he said, "I feel cured already." These comments were so rewarding for me. The couple even played a country-blues song together with the patient on the guitar and his girlfriend singing.

I guess all musicians feel in their heart that music is therapeutic without having any knowledge about music therapy. Not many patients have a background in music, but those who do seem to be open to music therapy. Some people are quick to get the idea of what music therapy is about and some people require more explanation. I have encountered several patients who already were familiar with music therapy. Those are the people who had been visited by our team previously or people who work in health care settings in which music therapy is provided.

The chance of encountering those people is rare. I realize that a part of our mission working at the hospitals is to educate and spread knowledge about music therapy.

CHAPTER 5: QUESTIONS FOR GROWTH

1. The title of this chapter is "The Elevator Pitch."
   Write down a pitch that you will use to advocate
   music therapy in "the elevator" in 30 seconds or less.
   Practice!

2. Why isn't music therapy for everyone? Give some
   examples of candidates that are not 'ideal' for music
   therapy services.

3. Explain an experience you have had with a client
   where the outcome was not easily observed. What do
   you believe happened? Was there something you could
   have done differently?

4. Observing limited responses from a patient can be
   tough. If you have a session where your patient
   remains asleep, what would you document in the
   medical chart?

5. In the second excerpt of this chapter, the therapist
   weighed both sides of the coin; music therapy through
   someone who understands it, and through someone
   who does not understand it. Take a second and do the
   same thing.

6. Witnessing a fight between patients right before a
   session starts can change the energy level of the room.
   What are some ways that you can clear your mind of
   it, then redirect the energy for clients in attendance?

CHAPTER 6 - WE ARE FAMILY: SUPPORT THROUGH MUSIC

> *"There is great comfort and inspiration in the feeling of close human relationships – a powerful force, to overcome the 'tough breaks,' which are certain to come to most of us from time to time."*
>
> *–Walt Disney*

A DAUGHTER'S FACILITATION

Mother with Thyroid Cancer

I went to the hospital and marched down the hall with my guitar and my cart. I got information from the charts, pulled my cart into a room, and discovered that I had no music. All of the books that belong in my cart were gone. "It's alright, I'm flexible," I told myself.

Once I was organized, I entered a middle-aged woman's room, prepared to try something different. I got out the marimba, and although she was hesitant, she said she would try it. She began telling me that she had been in and out of the hospital for the past year and a half and "now lung cancer is the problem even though I've never smoked." I said we could work on some relaxation and ways that she could cope with her hospital stays. She agreed but said she wanted me to wait for her daughter to return. She told me that she was never left alone; her family cares a great deal about her and always wants to surround her with love and support.

When her daughter returned, I thought that I might be able to facilitate some sharing between them. I asked the daughter if she would play the marimba with me. She did so without hesitation. "Think of a place that you would like to go with your mother and take her on a trip through listening to the instrument," I told the younger woman. Both the mother and daughter were able to share their imagery with one another and describe the experience they had through the musical improvisation. Music created a bond and offered the patient's family support during a long-term stay.

LOVE ALL AROUND
Grandfather with Prostate Cancer

I first saw this hospice patient when his granddaughter was present. He was lying in bed with his eyes closed, mostly nonresponsive while his granddaughter gave him a play-by-play of what was happening: "Two pretty girls are here to sing, grandpa!" Occasionally, he would moan in response to his granddaughter's words, but he kept his eyes closed. He would also reposition his body, reaching for the bedrails and slowly move his legs for several seconds until finally releasing and relaxing his body.

The man remained mostly still during the songs. I sang a few of the granddaughter's requests as well as some that she thought he would know. She told us that he was the one who always sang at all the parties. "He is a ladies' man, the charming one." As we were leaving, we said goodbye to the patient, and before we walked out the door, he surprisingly opened his eyes and extended his right arm straight up into the air, gesturing goodbye. The granddaughter was ecstatic. She thanked us and told us that he had experienced enough stimulation for the time being.

After a couple of hours, eight of the patient's family members arrived. His son-in-law stopped us in the hallway and requested that we see the man again. All ten of us gathered around the patient and started singing some of the family's favorites. The patient's eight-year-old great-grandson requested "I've Been Working on the Railroad" and he played an egg shaker along to the song.

> **LESSONS LEARNED**
>
> *"Music offers comfort, knowing that family is surrounding you with their own individual sounds, altogether as a cohesive group, a community."*

As we sang through the songs, the family members openly expressed their emotions; they cried, they hugged one another, they spoke positively to the patient. As we all surrounded him and sang, I told him that his family was surrounding him with comfort, love, and support. We sang and hummed through "You Are My Sunshine" and his daughter began to cry. Throughout all of the songs, the family members went from crying to laughing, to reminiscing, and to crying again. One family member expressed her sincere gratitude and told us that

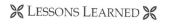

our services were necessary in the hospice setting. She said, "We couldn't have done this without you. Thank you."

From my experiences at hospice and in my own family, music is necessary when a family is together. Music binds. Music unites. Music evokes raw emotion.

NOT ALWAYS FOR THE PATIENT
Hospital Sibling and a Child with Autism

Feeling like I am giving the best music therapy possible is sometimes difficult when I'm working in pediatrics. Often, working with particular site, I have little knowledge about a patient's medical history and/or diagnosis. So much of my sessions are a constant state of assessment; this can be draining.

Just as we were leaving, two children interested in music were hanging out in the playroom; we decided to stay. One little guy sat next to me and looked like he wanted to play something. I asked him his favorite kind of music and was surprised when he said he liked jazz (the "old, good kind") and R&B. I put a drum in front of him and we started jamming. He then said, "How about you give me your best beat on guitar and I'll give you my best beat on drums, and we'll put them together. It will be amazing!"

We played for a little longer, and then I started doing a blues progression, and he jumped in by adding words. He sang about how he was bored and had to stay inside, he didn't like being away from home, and there's nothing to do while his brother was in the hospital. He clearly needed an outlet for creative expression and an opportunity to do something he liked. We all had a great time hanging out in the playroom and I loved what he brought to our session.

Energized, we returned to see another child, listed as a 12-year-old boy with autism. We didn't know for sure why he was in the hospital or the severity of his diagnosis, but I was excited to work with this client because of my past experience with this population. His disability was fairly profound, and he was nonverbal. We found him listening to headphones and hitting a toy while rocking back and forth. He seemed open to music therapy and became more involved and increasingly interactive as the session progressed. He began making more direct eye contact as we played drums and other instruments. Eventually, he took off the headphones and traded them for instruments so he could play with us. His mother looked on as he positively responded to music and at the end of our session we told her ways she may be able to get music therapy for him.

Goals for sessions are so important, even if they need to be changed during the session. Music therapists need as much information as possible regarding the reason for the referral to create an environment for therapy.

A FAMILY AFFAIR
Hospice Patient with Chronic Renal Failure

When I entered the referred patient's room, I first went to her roommate to ask if she would like music therapy. Her roommate declined services, saying that she was getting ready to leave.

Several family members surrounded the referred patient. She was lying in bed and unresponsive. Before I even reached their side of the room, one family member said that they would like some music. I leaned down and placed my hand on the patient's shoulder and told her who we were and why we were there. I explained that her family members and I were going to play some music for her. The family selected songs and joined in singing along.

I learned the patient was referred to as "Mother" by the whole family. We continued to sing and the most amazing thing happened. She opened her eyes for a few seconds. The family got quite excited and said, "Did you see that? She opened her eyes. I knew she could hear us! She knows!" The patient's attempt to look toward us was an awesome moment.

After a while, I began to sing an improvised song about Mother. I had never done this before and I don't know where the urge came from, but it felt right at that moment. I sang softly about the patient, how she seemed like a special woman, and how there was so much love around her. A few of the family members started to cry.

I continued to play the guitar and asked the family a few things that they would remember about the patient. One said, "Baseball." We learned about the patient's love/hate relationship with her home team and how she was a huge fan of the sport. I added in a few lines about her and her love of baseball before ending the song. I had kept the melody and lyrics simple in case any of the family members decided to sing along.

At the end of the song, I repeated her name over and over and said, "Oh Mother, we love you so." Just as I had hoped, the patient's granddaughter held the patient's hand, stroked her hair, and sang along with me. The family said, "That was so nice."

Her family began to express their appreciation and thanks for the music. One family member said, "I was just sitting here thinking, what a wonderful way to go. I felt like I was flying with her." Everyone in the room agreed it had been wonderful for them and the patient had enjoyed it.

The nurse then entered the room. She came in and looked at the patient and stated, "She looks more peaceful now, don't you think?" The family agreed and got excited as they told the nurse about the patient opening her eyes.

This session was particularly wonderful for me. I felt I had connected with the patient and her family. I believe that we allowed them to experience joy and sadness, in addition to sharing fond memories of their loved one. I was blown away by their comments and by the patient's soft gaze. I will never forget this family or the time that we spent with them.

CELEBRATION OF LIFE
Family of an Older Adult in Hospice Care

When I passed a hospice patient's room, he had five visitors. Normally, I do not hesitate to enter a room with family members, but the family seemed to be in deep conversation so I decided to try a few other rooms first. I went into the room across the hall from this resident, and while I was in there, I could see the five family members peek their heads into the room to hear what I was doing.

As I was getting ready to leave, I went out into the hallway to gather my belongings and begin to document. When I was putting my guitar away, I overheard them say, "Go ahead. Go ahead and talk to her." I wondered if they were talking about me. Sure enough, a few seconds later, one of the men came over and asked me if I only sang privately. I told him that I was there to provide services for the patients and families. He asked me if I could come in and sing for his family.

I entered the room, surprised to find that there were now eleven of the resident's family members in the room. The family all expressed their gratitude and excitement for me to be joining them. Luckily, I had some extra songbooks in my guitar case and distributed them to the family. The patient was lying in his bed, unresponsive. His family warned me that he would not respond or open his eyes. I explained the importance of touching and speaking to him. Walking over to the patient, I placed my hand on his shoulder and introduced myself. I told him, "I'm here to provide music with the help of your family, and I hope you will enjoy it. You must be a very special man because I've never seen this many people for a patient and felt so much love in one room."

Family members chose "Don't Get Around Much Anymore" and made joking comments to the patient. I instantly felt the mood lift in the room. Throughout the session, the family continued to share stories from the past and laughter filled the room. The last request was from one of the elderly ladies in the room. She requested the song "Twist and Shout."

When she made this request, everyone began to laugh. I instructed the family that I would sing and they could repeat to fill in the song. The family continued to giggle and sing. The woman who requested the song also jumped up and led everyone to the end of the song with the "Ah" section of the song. Even though the patient was unresponsive, I was sure that he could hear us and was sharing the joy with his family.

When the song was over, I nostalgically said goodbye to the patient and his delightful family and thanked them for the opportunity to share part of my day with them. As I left the room, I could hear the family laugh and joke with one another. Just as I was about to leave, one of the men in the room came running out after me. He said, "Thank you so much. We have spent so much time mourning. We really needed some joy and a little pick-me-up. Thank you for making us laugh and remember."

I was truly touched by this; I had to take a moment to think about how important this intervention was for the patient and his family. I left hospice that day with happiness in my heart and "Twist and Shout" stuck in my head.

A NEEDED RELEASE
Hospice Patient with Ovarian Cancer

I have had many moving interventions throughout the course of working with hospice patients, but this one exceeded all of them. Shortly after arriving at the facility, a hospice nurse informed me that a woman had recently been admitted. She said she thought that the patient would be interested in music therapy. I always appreciate getting referrals from nurses, so I eagerly set down my belongings.

Upon entering the patient's room, I was stopped by another nurse, who asked if she could make a quick bed change. As I waited for the nurse to finish, one of the patient's visitors came out into the hallway and stood next to me. I immediately noticed the resemblance between this woman and the patient. She said they were sisters and that they had grown to look more like each other over the years. She told me that her sister had always been a strong woman, but that her fight was over and she was prepared to die. We talked about the importance of acceptance; she assured me several times that her sister was ready to welcome the next life. Apparently, it had been a long and tiring battle.

The nurse came into the hallway and asked us back into the room. I introduced myself to the patient, her sister, and her daughter. I explained what music therapy was and what I could offer; shortly after, another music therapist arrived. I was confident that we could offer this family something meaningful.

The patient stated she wasn't experiencing any pain or anxiety. She quickly scanned the table of contents of the songbook and began naming song after song that she wanted to hear. The first song she requested was "Amazing Grace." Although this song is requested so often, I always find it interesting to observe the reactions of those listening. The song means something different to everyone; I think that's what makes it so special.

Next she asked to hear "I Can See Clearly Now." The patient's sister and daughter looked thoughtfully at her while the patient looked over the words. About halfway through the song, the patient's eyes began to well up with tears. I felt myself wanting to comfort her, but I knew that the people that she needed most were right next to her. Very little was said after this second song. The patient then requested "I Will Remember You" and turned to her family. She said, "Come over here. Come sit close to me, right on the bed." Her family crowded around on her hospital bed and squeezed her tightly.

The lyrics were, "I will remember you, will you remember me? Don't let your life pass you by, weep not for the memories." Once my hands struck the guitar and began to play, her daughter and sister began to cry. When the other music therapist and I came in with the words, the tears fell harder. The confidence and assurance that the patient's sister had given me in the hallway suddenly turned to grief, fear, and sadness. As the family held each other tightly and cried, it felt as if strong energy covered every inch of the room.

When the song had come to an end, the patient looked at us and said, "Thank you so much, ladies. This is exactly what we needed." I shall never forget the image of this family on the tiny hospital bed, sharing their love and tears with one another.

LIKE FATHER, LIKE SON
Young Adult's Recovery from a Car Accident

I had several interactions with a referred patient and his father. The first visit was a little intimidating, as the patient's song selection consisted of Korn, Nine Inch Nails, and some other heavy rock bands I wasn't prepared to play. We had a brief conversation about Metallica before his father entered the room. His father was excited to see us and named some classic rock selections that his son also liked. After playing some Pink Floyd and Lynyrd Skynyrd, the patient became more restful. He seemed to have dozed off a bit during the music and commented that he had been having difficulty resting. This was the first time he felt able to sleep, so we left him to rest for the afternoon. I promised I would learn some Metallica and visit again soon.

For the next visit, the patient had been moved to another room. He complained of pain and seemed irritable. Once again, his father welcomed me. He told me that he is a sound engineer and works behind the scenes at rock concerts, often accompanied by his son. Their lives revolved around music and because of this, his son liked a variety of genres.

I began one of the Metallica ballads I had learned. Not long into the first song, the patient reached out his hand to touch mine as I was strumming and said dreamily, "It's so beautiful. This is the first time I've actually understood the words." During the next song, his father walked to the corner of the room, and I could hear him softly sniffing.

The patient asked me to keep playing because it relaxed him and helped him sleep.

His father told me more about their life and how once, when his son was a toddler, he snuck on stage to play the drums after a concert. He said he was always listening to music - even while he slept. When I left, his father hugged me. The patient was alone and appeared to be sleeping soundly for the following session. I didn't want to bother him and went to get a "Sorry I missed you" card from my cart. In the meantime, his father arrived and asked me to come into the room. The patient was very groggy and didn't respond when his dad asked if he wanted music; however, moments later the patient said quietly, "Don't leave me alone."

The father told me how much yesterday's visit had meant to him and his son; that his son slept peacefully for the entire afternoon after I left. I played a few songs that his dad requested. In between songs, he would talk to me about his son and their life together. The dad said, "It might not seem like it, but he is hearing this." He sat vigilantly by his son. His concern and emotion was apparent. For this session, it was the father who needed the music the most. His father opened up to me that the patient had lost his girlfriend in the car accident. His father was behind them and witnessed the accident. On this last visit, the father said that their faith would be the main thing to get them through, but that music would be the other healing tool.

Oftentimes, music therapy is just as important for the family as it is to the patient ... the father needed this visit. Being fully present is so important for patients like this and their family members—those who recognize that, for them, music will be the thing to help them cope and deal with their experience.

Take a Breath
Patient Recovery from Post-Pacemaker Implant

This patient had been experiencing abnormally slow heart rhythms and, as a result, had surgery to implant a pacemaker. Now recovering from her operation, the woman was experiencing generalized weakness. She was expected to return to rehab for occupational and physical therapy when she regained her strength.

When I met the patient's daughter, she seemed a bit on edge and frustrated. She mentioned to me that the rehab team had stressed her mother's need for deep breathing exercises because her current breathing was far too shallow. Her daughter seemed quite adamant about this. I explained that I could assist her mother with some deep breathing techniques.

I waited a few minutes before entering the patient's room to give her and her daughter a few minutes of privacy. When I entered, the patient was sitting in her chair, looking quite full of life and saying, "I'm quite ready for a sing-along." At her request, I pulled out the songbook and let her pick some songs. After we sang the song "Country Roads," I could sense agitation in the daughter. She kept looking at the clock and trying to rush the singing process by saying things like, "OK, let's go," and cutting the conversations short.

I suggested we try some deep breathing techniques. At this request, the daughter immediately relaxed and began to talk with her mother about the rehab team's suggestions and the importance of deep breathing. From there, I lead them through a deep breathing exercise, including some tips and pointers as well as music and imagery exercises. I immediately noticed the energy in the room change; the daughter needed to stop and breathe almost as much as the patient.

We discussed deep breathing and the mind/body connection for about ten minutes. I told the patient that she could use these techniques to help her sleep, calm her mind, and renew and refresh her whole body. She seemed excited about the possibilities and mentioned that she used to do yoga, but had forgotten about the benefits of deep breathing. After our short relaxation session, we ended with "What a Wonderful World," at the patient's request.

LIONS INTO LAMBS
Support for a Patient with Multiple Diagnoses

Based on notes from case managers, nurses, and other health care professionals, this patient appeared to experience nausea due to chemotherapy. The record also indicated psychosocial issues involving anger directed toward family members, especially where the patient's husband was concerned. I read multiple progress notes, including statements such as "patient verbally abusive to husband."

Once outside, my co-therapist and I realized that the patient had many family members present, which was intriguing considering progress notes regarding family interactions. The patient was sitting on the side of her bed while her son fed her an early dinner. I immediately got the feeling that this was a woman with spunk.

I introduced myself and began to ask the patient if she would like some music therapy. As soon as the word music came out of my mouth, she said "Music? Oh, we love music. I played saxophone, clarinet, and piano." After coming to the conclusion that the children's songs being requested by the patient and her grandsons were not in our current repertoire, she said, "Play whatever you have." We decided to play something upbeat, to which the kids could drum and shake along.

The patient was hooting and hollering, the daughter-in-law was smiling, and the patient's husband was singing occasionally. Her husband requested "Besame Mucho," during which the patient and her husband got even closer. The patient said, "Kiss me, kiss me a lot" to her husband, and they both began to cry. The couple spent moments verbalizing tenderly to each other.

I looked at the faces around the room. The grandchildren seemed to realize this music was not "fun," but the older boy had a peaceful expression. The daughter-in-law held her child as she smiled and swayed to the music. Although the patient's son was concerned about keeping his mother covered at all times, his expression seemed a little less anguished.

As we prepared to leave, the patient said, "This is what patients need. You made my day."

CHAPTER 6: QUESTIONS FOR GROWTH

1.   These excerpts demonstrate therapeutic approaches to music therapy when family members are present. Is it ever appropriate to ask that the family to leave you alone with the patient for one-on-one therapy? In the excerpt, "A Needed Release," how was the experience enhanced for the patient therapeutically with the family members present?

2.   Seeing a room full of family members can be intimidating or uncomfortable. How might you give a delivery for music therapy to such a room of people?

3.   In what ways is songwriting with family members a way for them to build connection with the patient?

4.   During a session, one of the therapists began to improvise a song to the patient. Perhaps you are able to do this; perhaps you need practice in this area. What are some good ways to practice improvisation?

5.   One of the therapists from this chapter greeted a patient even when his family insisted he could not hear her. Was it necessary for the therapist to greet the patient?

Chapter 7 · Those Fragile Moments

"No one wants to die. Even people who want to go to heaven don't want to die to get there. And yet, death is the destination we all share. No one has ever escaped it. And that is as it should be, because death is very likely the single best invention of life. It is life's change agent — it makes room for the new."

— Steve Jobs

A Change of Heart

A Family's Last Hours

A nurse approached me and said that one particular room needed music therapy; however, most likely, would decline services. The patient only had a few hours to live. The patient's daughter and son were present at her bedside.

I passed the daughter in the hallway as she was walking to get some water. I asked if she would care for some music. She said nicely that she was fine with the CD player in the room. I lingered with violin in hand — wanting to ask the patient myself.

I watched the daughter's face lift a bit as she spotted my violin. I told her, "I am here to provide music therapy" and offered a few different interventions. I also told her that I had spent the past week with her mom and really enjoyed her sweetness. The daughter was listening intently and asked me to come by later.

When I entered the patient's room, the patient (their mother) was taking in her last hours of air. She had the characteristic traits of a person actively passing: body lying on the bed, labored and erratic breathing, mouth open, eyes closed and unresponsive. I began playing relaxing music in the patient's favorite genre, Celtic. I had coincidentally listened to Irish music on the drive to the hospice facility and had that genre on my mind. After playing for a bit, the brother and sister looked more peaceful and smiled at their mother and me. I attempted to entrain the music with the patient's breath and hoped she knew the music was coming from people who love her. Her son was moved to tears and thanked me profusely for providing music for his mother.

I almost felt like an intercessory; the music seemed able to communicate to the patient from the children. I never know how the music will work. For me, the key is to be open to music's power and stepping out of its way. I offered the family peace and left the room.

MUSIC OF THE HEART
A Father and Daughter Share a Moment

A quick glance from the patient's doorway left me with the thought that death was near for him. He was lying flat on his back with his mouth gaped open and his eyes closed. Other patients were unavailable, so I unpacked my viola and went to his room. His daughter apprehensively allowed me to enter with the expectation of playing a few old tunes and then leave with a gentle smile. But between the time I entered and left, the room was filled with spirit and life - driven by music.

The patient was awake at this point and was sitting up slightly, supported by the bed, his big blue eyes open. He did not look directly at me, but always in my direction, listening to the music with a clearly positive affect. Then he asked me to play and sing at the same time. This was the first combination request I had ever had with voice and viola. I began to sing and play the sweet lullaby, "Edelweiss."

After I finished, the daughter and her father thanked me for the song. Then she said something that opened my eyes. She told her father that she wished that he could see me playing. The patient had lost his vision. He told his daughter, "Music flows and reaches the heart. I can feel your music and see your beauty."

The patient talked a little longer with me about love, music, listening, and seeing. His daughter tearfully shared that this was the first time that she heard her father talk so much since being admitted to hospice nearly two weeks prior. She said she was able to learn things about her father that she did not previously know. I learned to not forget the power of music to deliver and share life through sound.

A FAMILY ASSURED
Male with Multiple Cancers

I was referred to a male hospice patient diagnosed with liver, lung, and colon cancers; the patient was no longer responsive. We double-checked with the nurse that this was the referral that she wanted us to see. She told us that this was the correct patient and that he loved music.

There was music playing on a CD player in his room when we entered. I turned it off and looked at the CD cases nearby; a variety of classical music including hymns on classical guitar. His breathing was long and very audible. I looked at my watch to see the length of time between each breath: six seconds. I tried to match the tempo of the music to his breathing. I noticed a photograph on his board of three people on motorcycles and a cowboy hat next to his head.

After about 30 minutes, I said it was nice to meet him and I would be back next week. About an hour and a half went by while I visited other patients.

As I was getting ready to leave, I saw a man sitting in the lobby who looked like one of the men in the photograph. I asked him if he was the patient's son, and he said yes. I introduced myself as the music therapist and told him we had been in with his father.

I told him about the songs we sang, and he smiled at "Country Roads." He said a nurse had told him that we were the last ones to be in with his father.

A woman walked in with two younger children, and introduced herself as the patient's daughter. She said,

"Oh, music therapy. What do you do?" I told her that we had sung a few songs to her father and that I matched the tempo of the music to his breath. She said, "Oh, were you in there when he took his last breath?"

I did not know he had died. I said "No, but we were in there about an hour and a half ago." He must have passed shortly after we left. They smiled and thanked me. I hope the family was comforted knowing that we were there for their father. I also hope the music provided a peaceful bridge from this place to the next for the patient.

✂ LESSONS LEARNED ✂

"Hospice is a very fragile place. Even though the audience may not be responsive, those who are capable of the least may need it the most."

FIVE-FOOT-TWO
Reflecting on a Journey

My patient was a spunky 92-year-old woman, 5'2" with sharp blue eyes, smooth skin, and a head of silky white hair with glittery fire-red strands. I had been working with her since the beginning of my internship; we had wonderful moments together as well as some difficult days. I grew very fond of her.

Due to her shortness of breath, she was limited to singing one or two songs. When she didn't sing, she agreed to accompany me on the drum or other percussion instruments while I played my guitar or ukulele. Some of her favorite songs were "Five Foot Two," "He's Got the Whole World in His Hands," "Pearly Shells," and "With a Little Help from My Friends." She played like a champ. One day I showed her my maracas from Puerto Rico. She was having so much fun that she got carried away in playing along with me to "Twist and Shout" that one of the staff members had to give her breathing medicine under her tongue. Oh, how we laughed that day.

The woman often talked about how much she and her husband used to love to dance and about their travel experiences. One day, she asked me how old I was, and when I told her, she replied, "My dear, we have 70 years between us. That certainly is a beautiful thing!"

During our last month together, I dealt with some emotions due to my attachment to this patient. I struggled with the idea of letting go. The day after she passed away, I arrived at her door with no idea that her room would be empty. As I turned the corner, I anticipated the possibility of her not being there. A staff member told me that she had passed away the previous morning. To my surprise, a happy, peaceful feeling came over me. No tears, only a grin from ear to ear filled my face. She was now in a special place—dancing with her son and husband.

Working with this patient made me more comfortable with embracing death as a part of life. I have learned a lot about myself including how much I enjoy working in hospice care. It is emotionally challenging, but filled with many beautiful hair-raising and tearful moments that I feel fortunate to share with the patients and their families during the last days of their lives.

Solemnly Solitary

A Woman Facing End of Life Alone

The patient was lying in bed. Her progress notes mentioned multiple times that she was unresponsive, but that didn't prepare me for what I found. Last week, the woman had accepted services verbally, but I was not the therapist who saw her. I offered music therapy to her and asked her to blink to indicate she wanted us to stay. I am not sure if she blinked or not, but because of her previous acceptance, I stayed.

I sang soft, soothing songs like "Amazing Grace," "Love Me Tender," and "Somewhere Over the Rainbow." I knelt down beside the bed while the patient lay there gasping for breath.

She looked like what I imagine death to look like. She was, in my opinion, actively dying or very close to it. One of her arms was completely purple. I reached my arm out to stroke the other arm. She appeared fragile; I hoped I wasn't hurting her though I was barely touching her. At times while I was singing, the patient made slight vocalizations, but I have no way of knowing if she was trying to sing or if she was uncomfortable and still gasping for more breath. I don't recall ever making eye contact with her. I do not think I was avoiding eye contact, but I felt like she was looking over into space.

> **Lessons Learned**
>
> *"As therapists, we must process our own thoughts and feelings. Pushing them down does not make them disappear."*

I thought to myself: before I came, she was alone. When I left fifteen minutes later, she was alone again. I kept thinking how lonely it must be there with no family or loved ones. I wondered if she was thirsty or needed some balm for her lips. I hoped someone else would come see her and be with her when she died. At the time, I was unaffected. I noticed her isolation, but I took it at face value as the way things work. Thinking about it now, I just swallowed and avoided those feelings. When I went to bed that night, I cried for her.

As therapists, we must process our own thoughts and feelings; pushing them down does not make them disappear.

THE WORLD STOOD STILL
A Shared Experience Among Strangers

Upon entering the patient's room, I was struck by how exhausted she appeared. She lay in the quiet light of mid-morning as though she had wrestled with sleeplessness for many nights. I immediately reached for her hand, spoke in a calm voice, and asked if she would like to hear some relaxing music. She slowly opened her eyes and nodded her head ever so slightly. As I strummed my guitar, I was overcome with feelings of helplessness. She appeared to be in such pain and all I could offer were a few simple chords. How could I help this woman? I tried to remind myself to breathe, but I stood there feeling so small.

A chaplain, his assistant, and an individual I assumed to be a family member joined me. I waited patiently while they introduced themselves to the patient. Immediately following this, the chaplain requested "Amazing Grace" and without a moment's hesitation, I handed lyric sheets to everyone in the room. As we began to sing, the room filled with a deep resonance that sent chills up my spine. Everything came into focus and I felt the power of song. Each individual showed their deep caring for this human in immense suffering by expressing their feelings through music. We all gave the patient the most vital of all things needed for survival: love.

We finished with "How Great Thou Art" and a brief prayer. It dawned on me that the patient had been crying for some time through closed eyes. I reached out and offered my hand in goodbye and she took it, looked into my eyes and whispered, "Thank you." I became aware of all the sounds of the hospital filling the space around me as I left the room. I understood what an important service we had offered. No medical technology, however advanced, could provide the kind of solace found in simple song.

This was my first musical experience with someone who appeared to be so close to death. While I feel such a deep sense of importance regarding what was shared during the intervention, it is difficult to explain it in objective terms. It is also difficult to communicate the importance of such interventions in the rational, scientific language that dominates our health care system. How can we bridge this language barrier? I am still unsure.

SHARING A PRECIOUS MOMENT
Cancer Patient and His Daughter

The patient demonstrated passive listening and remained unresponsive throughout the session. His breathing pattern was heavy, and he showed signs of agitation as evidenced by loud noises with each inhale and occasional thrashing motions of the neck and head.

The man's daughter informed me and my co-therapist of her father's preferred music and gave specific song choices including, "Let It Be," "Hey Jude," and "Bridge Over Troubled Water." My co-therapist played the guitar and sang while I added harmonies. The daughter held her father's hand, touching his face and crying. She shared stories about her father's youth and some of his accomplishments with his choir. She told us that these song choices held emotional significance within their father-daughter relationship. As the session came to a close, the daughter said, "Music will always be welcome." The patient's breathing had softened and his agitation had diminished. About five minutes later, a nurse approached us and said that the patient had just passed.

The fact that this patient passed away moments after our session was humbling to me. Emotional control was difficult during that session. I discovered that I was greatly moved by and sensitive to the father-daughter relationship during these powerful final moments of his life. I understood more deeply the importance of what we do as music therapists in regards to the end-of-life transition. By providing songs that the patient and his daughter connected to, we created a peaceful environment for the patient in his last moments. I realized, to share such personal moments, how strong, open, and trusting his daughter must be.

During the session, I kept thinking of my own father. I wondered whether I would be comfortable enough to share the room with a stranger in such an intimate moment. This is when I realized how much of an honor it was to share this time with her. It is truly a gift when family members of hospice patients share their loved one's final moments with a music therapist.

THE EMPTY ROOM

Supporting a Daughter through a Mother's Decline

When we received a referral for this patient, I had seen her previously on another floor. The referral was disheartening to me because it came by family request after the patient moved under hospice care and was at the hospital with a morphine drip.

I provided treatment to the patient while her daughter was in the room. She stroked her mother's shoulder and held her hand as I sang the patient's preferred music. At this point, the patient was still coherent, making eye contact with me occasionally. Her breathing was labored, but when I asked her, "Is the music helping you relax?" she nodded and whispered, "Yes," through her breathing mask. She occasionally drifted off. By the end of the session, the patient had fallen asleep and the daughter thanked me for coming.

I told the daughter that I would follow up throughout the course of this following week. She said, "I don't know if she will be here in a week," and began to cry. We stepped into the hallway, and she told me that her mother had decided not to undergo any more treatments because they had been unsuccessful. They knew the patient was going to die, but they didn't know when. The daughter was tearful, and I offered our services to her at any time, stating that we often provide support when it comes time for end-of-life care. I told her we'd try our best to be available at any time and that she can put an "urgent" status on the request if needed.

A few days later, I went to follow up with the patient and her daughter. The patient was in bed, non-responsive, and her breathing was severely labored. The daughter was by her mother's bed- side, tears streaming down her face. She greeted me with a smile and welcomed me. She requested several of her mother's favorites and we sang to her. The daughter was crying during the entire session. She told me that the last time her mother had been awake was "during the music yesterday, and she was able to tell you that it was helping her, so that was very special. She's not awake anymore, but I know she can hear it and it is helping her now." I validated the daughter, telling her that the sense of hearing is one of the last senses to go and that

I was confident that her mother could hear her voice and the music, and that it was comforting to her.

The next day, I went to check in with the patient and daughter, preparing myself for the idea that the mother could be in an even worse condition. I saw nothing but an empty sterile room as I was walking down the hallway toward where she had been. My heart sank. Immediately, I thought of her daughter - this precious woman who had just lost her mother. I wish I could have been there to help her during that difficult moment, but I am glad that I was able to help her in some way while her mother was still here.

I feel honored to provide the smallest comfort through music while someone is dying and their family members are hurting. In these situations, the work is so meaningful and special to the family—and to the therapists.

LET GO
A Family Says Goodbye

As I was singing for a patient on one side of the room, I noticed and overheard a minister blessing the patient on the other side of the curtain. After the minister left, I overheard a young woman say, "Mom, do you hear the lovely music?"

After I finished my session with the first patient, I peeked over to offer music. The daughter said, "We would love music." She asked me if I knew "Somewhere My Love" from the movie *Dr. Zhivago* and I did, because that was my grandpa's favorite song.

The patient was positioned on her back, her head facing toward the left, and she was making gurgling sounds. About thirty seconds into singing, the patient stopped making the gurgling sounds, she became more at ease. Her daughter and two other relatives sat nearby, with tears in their eyes. I could tell that these were going to be the patient's last moments due to her pale, white skin and her eyes staring off into space. I offered the family a choice of religious songs and they picked "How Great Thou Art." During this song, the daughter was at her mother's side, holding her hand, and she was reassuring her mother, "It is alright to go to heaven."

The mother passed. I continued to play "How Great Thou Art," just humming the melody and then transitioned into "Amazing Grace." Once the nurse came in to the room to verify the patient had passed, she thanked me for the music. Several minutes later, we all had to leave the room. The daughter hugged and thanked me saying, "It was meant to be." The family members recalled how much the patient loved music and said, "The music helped her (the patient) to let go."

I had witnessed how powerful music is; after only thirty seconds, the patient was comforted by the music. I was so glad that I was there for this moment because it was meaningful for me as well. I felt honored to be a part of the journey.

PURE BEAUTY
Looking Past the Disease

Walking into the patient's room, I felt as though I was looking at the face of death. It sounds so awful to say, but she looked like a skeleton lying in bed. She was so pale and thin, only a few strands of hair on her head, skin peeling from her scalp and face, her eyes sunken.

I was told by the nurse that she may or may not open her eyes, but to introduce myself and play for her anyway.

When I introduced myself, I saw the patient move her left hand, although she did not open her eyes. I went over to the other side and took her left hand in mine, explaining I was there to play relaxing music for her. She squeezed my hand tightly, eyes still closed. I began improvising on a chord before beginning a song. The patient turned her head toward me, opened her eyes slightly and said, "I like that." I told her I was so happy to be playing for her and all she needed to do was listen and relax. She closed her eyes again and I sang "Edelweiss."

To my astonishment, she began to hum along with me. Her affect became soft and relaxed with a slight smile on her face as she hummed. I told her I loved hearing her sing and thought she had a beautiful voice. I chose several more songs, and she hummed along to almost every one. Occasionally, she would open her eyes and smile at me. After one song, she said, "This brings back many memories." I asked her, "Good memories?" She smiled and said, "Oh, yes."

Watching her enjoy the music, I felt as though I was looking straight past this woman's disease and into her beautiful soul. She was radiating beauty as she hummed. I thought about what this woman may have done and seen in her lifetime and how amazing it was to be at her bedside as she was nearing the end of her life. I felt honored to meet this beautiful person, and fought back tears as she hummed along with "My Wild Irish Rose."

As I played "Que Sera, Sera," she opened her eyes wide, lifted her head towards me, and sang the entire song with me – she never once closed her eyes. When the song was over, she quietly said, "Thank you," laid her head back down, and closed her eyes again. Almost instantly, her respiration deepened and she began to fall asleep. I took her hand in mine and told her it was a pleasure to sing with her today. She did not open her eyes, but repeated, "Thank you, thank you,"

✂ LESSONS LEARNED ✂

"I know that dealing with death is emotional and difficult, but it can also be inspiring and extremely touching."

several times. Leaving her room, I felt that I had seen the beauty of life rather than the face of death. My heart was full of joy, sadness, honor, empathy, and respect for this beautiful woman. I can hardly explain the unique experience of her soul and the sweetness of the touch from her wrinkled hand.

As Long as You Need Me
Finding the Joy in End-of-Life Support

A nurse approached me in the ICU and referred a patient who was actively dying; his family had requested music therapy. Upon seeing the distraught look on this nurse's face, I decided to momentarily forgo the charting for my last patient until after I had seen the newly referred patient and his family.

I entered the small room to find eight people seated. The patient was lying in bed, alarms constantly buzzing, signaling that his vital signs were beginning to drop. As I crossed the room to better position myself to see everyone in the room, I noticed two children sitting on the far side of the room on the floor, huddled together and weeping.

There was an air of tension in the room, although I was greeted with warm smiles. The family asked for soothing instrumental music. I improvised on guitar for some time and then heard the patient's sister softly humming along with the chords I played. I asked them what songs were special to the patient. The family settled on some inspirational songs and sang "Amazing Grace" as I played. The patient's wife was called out of the room by a social worker, causing the daughter to cry so hard she could barely breathe; her aunt had to take her out of the room. The men in the family discussed with me the patient's favorite types of music as I continued to softly strum my guitar.

The patient's daughter and sister entered the room again. My fingers hurt quite badly at this point, since I had been playing constantly for forty-five minutes; however, I told the family I could stay as long as they wanted. When the patient's son indicated that he wanted me to stay, I momentarily left the room and brought back the lap marimba, which I demonstrated for the children. The oldest son modeled playing it for his younger siblings. The three younger children took turns playing as I accompanied them on guitar, trying to reflect the music they were making.

An amazing thing happened. The children smiled. All of them, one by one, began to smile and enjoy making music. They talked and laughed and remembered things about their father that seemed almost forgotten after seeing his heart rate and blood pressure steadily drop for the last few hours. The smiles on the children's faces became infectious. Everyone was smiling and talking again, something they had not done since I had entered the room nearly an hour earlier. The patient's brother even played the marimba briefly, stating that the sound of the instrument was relaxing to him.

I sensed that it was time for me to make my exit. The atmosphere of the room had changed drastically in ninety minutes. A room originally filled with sadness and tension was now filled with love and fond remembrance of a loved one.

FINDING THE GOOD
A Mother Recently Diagnosed with Terminal Cancer

I recognized a patient's name from a different floor. When I stopped to see her, we joked briefly that she must have been getting better since she was now closer to the front door. She told me she was starting chemotherapy and that she would very much like music. However, she wanted to wait until her family came back so they could enjoy it together.

I came back to her room about an hour later and found the patient, her daughter, and her future son-in-law helping her get ready to use the restroom. As we waited, I spoke with the patient's daughter about her mother's prognosis. She informed me that only seventeen days ago her mother was diagnosed with terminal cancer, which completely shocked the family since the patient was only admitted for back pain. The hospital pastoral staff had helped the patient come to terms with her illness and convinced her to attempt chemotherapy to enable her to live at least a few extra months. Lastly, she told me how her mother's eyes lit up when she talked about our session.

The patient returned to her bed and the family insisted I sit down to play, since they all had chairs. I sat facing the patient's bed, where she was lying comfortably. She suggested that each person take a turn selecting songs. As we went around the room, each person added a personal story to explain why they had chosen each song. Her future son-in-law even dedicated "Somewhere Over the Rainbow" to 'the best mother-in-law in the whole world.' A nurse came in to remove the patient's IV drip and stated that she thought all patients receiving chemotherapy should have music therapy. The patient and her family agreed heartily. The patient thanked me for coming to see her again and we spoke briefly about her discharge plan.

The first thing I thought after hearing that this patient had terminal cancer was, "Why do all my favorite patients have to die?" I had some time to think about this and realized that even though these people are in my life only a short time, each one of them is so special. Not only do I give something to them, they also give me something in return: the gift of themselves. I am lucky to have spent time with her and her beautiful family.

CHAPTER 7: QUESTIONS FOR GROWTH

1. List five religious and five secular songs that music therapists should add to their repertoire for hospice and/or end of life.

2. Death can be difficult to comprehend and to prepare for; whether you're a music therapist, a patient, or a family member. As a music therapist, do you feel that you can handle the therapeutic responsibilities in the death and grieving population? Do you feel that you can stay grounded? How can you prepare yourself for hospice work while being present with the patient?

3. When a patient is said to be unresponsive, what are some ways that you can check for possible response from the patient during a session? How can you use the music to check for stimulation with the patient? What is the importance of still communicating to a hospice patient even if they're unresponsive?

4. The therapist in "Solemnly Solitary" was unsure how to objectively write her experiences with a patient. She ended her excerpt from this chapter by asking, "How can we bridge this language barrier," the language barrier between experiences and objective/scientific writing. Any ideas?

5. How can music-making with family serve as a catalyst for emotional release?

6. HIPAA states that the patient always has the right to refuse music therapy services, however, we are trained to reinforce and motivate clients, even if they initially refuse. How can we tell what the limit is while encouraging and reinforcing the behavior outcomes the treatment team wants to see from a patient? How do we know when we've gone far enough?

CHAPTER 8 - HELP ME HELP YOU: WORKING WITH OTHERS

"In the long history of humankind, those who learned to collaborate and improvise most effectively have prevailed."

–Charles Darwin

AN URGENT CALL
A Nurse and a Surgical ICU (SICU) Patient

As I poured over a chart at the nurses' station in the SICU, I heard someone behind me say, "Music therapy! We need music in here!" I was somewhat startled but happy that my services were being requested, so I turned around and entered the room from which the nurse called.

The nurse informed me that her patient was in a great deal of pain. I indicated that I could work with him after seeing my scheduled patient. The patient said he could wait, but the nurse pressed forward, explaining that her patient was in a lot of pain and asked if I could see him immediately. I realized this was an instance in which I had to assign priority based on immediate need.

I grabbed my guitar and asked the patient what kind of music he preferred. He said he liked all music and that he used to play the guitar. The urgency was palpable, especially as I observed the grimaces on the patient's face and the accompanying concern of his nurse. After finding a song and asking for a self-report of pain from the patient, I began to play. The nurse held the songbook in front of me with one hand, comforted her patient with the other, and sang along at every opportunity. The intervention began to work; the patient grimaced less, closed his eyes, hummed along at times, and smiled occasionally.

As the nurse and I noticed the apparent changes in the patient, she smiled and nodded at me. I slowed the tempo in hopes that the music would no longer stimulate motor movement. As I did this, the patient actually fell asleep.

As I quietly gathered my things and thanked the nurse, the patient slowly awakened and expressed his appreciation. I asked about his pain level and he said, "Minus forty." I smiled broadly and told him to let his nurse or doctor know if he wanted a music therapy follow-up.

❧ LESSONS LEARNED ❧

"In caring for patients, we must always remember the team members, communicate with them whenever appropriate, and hear their communication in return."

This was an amazing experience. The nurse's obvious faith in the power of music therapy and her strong emotional support and encouragement edified the intervention, which I believe influenced an incredible outcome. I feel enormous gratitude to the music and the nurse who knew it was just what her patient needed.

STRESS BUSTER
Group Session with RNs

"Where's my big drum?" asked a nurse when I appeared in the nurses' station on my floor.

"I've got your drum; it's waiting for you in the nurses' lounge. Come on, let's go!" I said.

After this initial playful conversation, the charge nurse and nurse educator prompted all of the nurses to go to the music therapy group. Having nurses follow me down the hall made me feel like the pied piper. What fun!

The first group of the in-service was high energy. At least ten nurses in the room all made a lot of noise. We gave them a steady energetic pulse, guided them through dynamic changes, and encouraged them to release their voices during the session. This did not take much encouragement, as the hooting and hollering certainly could be heard down the hall. After dynamics, we facilitated instrument sculpting and most of the nurses understood the cues. We encouraged them to close their eyes and listen to the musical conversation. At the end of the session, everyone was laughing, smiling, chatting, and sweating.

The second group was slightly smaller and a more subdued than the first. The group consisted of all women and one man. The man took a laid-back approach to his music making, but he participated fully and followed cues well. One nurse really got into the experience, occasionally laughing and joking about her playing. Another nurse appeared uncomfortable with her musical ability as she tried several various instruments, but maintained a good sense of humor about the process.

In both groups, nurses encouraged, joked, and teased each other, which created an atmosphere of fun and acceptance. I had a wonderful time facilitating in the abbreviated but focused environment. After the groups, we received more referrals from nurses as they left and went back to work, demonstrating that showing someone the power that music therapy can elicit is worth a thousand words.

STARTING EARLY
Pre-Surgical Support for Couple

The census indicated several pre-surgery patients would arrive on the floor that morning. I saw a few patients in the pre-operation waiting areas, but the atmosphere was too hectic to do music therapy.

I tried to do an intervention with one patient, but he declined. I met one of the charge nurses for the first time and when I told her I was there to do music therapy, she was enthusiastic. She said the best time to come would be early morning, "They start arriving around 4:30 a.m."

The next day, I arrived early and met with the charge nurse. She made a list of patients who could benefit from music therapy and took me to a patient in one of the waiting areas. She approached the patient and asked if she wanted to receive music therapy while she waited for surgery. Initially, the patient was hesitant, but the charge nurse told her that music therapy helps patients relax before surgeries. The patient agreed, saying, "Oh yes, I'd like that."

We began with deep breathing and a relaxation exercise. The patient's husband arrived after a couple minutes and joined us. He sat next to his wife and held her hand. Initially, they both had their eyes open, but after a minute or two, they closed their eyes as they relaxed. After the exercise, they thanked me and said it helped them calm their nerves. The patient pointed out that the way the nurse presented music therapy to her made her open to it.

I realized through this experience that networking with staff is crucial, especially when starting a new program. This nurse is a great resource, especially since she believes music therapy benefits the patients.

Music Helps the Medicine Go Down
Receiving Positive Feedback from a Colleague

The physician referred this patient to music therapy for psychosocial support. When I entered the room, she welcomed me with a smile. We got to know each other and then discussed her music preferences. She was a pianist and enjoyed playing popular music. She also loved listening to classical music. I showed her my songbooks and she chose several songs.

We spoke between each song and soon the nurse came in to give the patient her medication. The woman looked somewhat anxious while the nurse was getting the medication ready. I began to play "Amazing Grace," a preferred song that the patient identified earlier when looking at the song list. As the nurse injected the pain medication, the patient focused on me the entire time. I kept singing until the nurse was finished, smiling at the patient reassuringly.

As the nurse finished, the patient said, "Well, that wasn't so bad. The music certainly helps the medication go down easier." We closed with one last song, then I asked the patient if she wanted a follow-up session; she smiled and said, "Yes, whenever you have some extra time." I told her I would bring the keyboard next time so we could play together.

As I was charting in the nurses' station, the patient's nurse approached me and said, "That was the brightest I have ever seen that patient. I just thought you should know."

A SPARKLING REFERRAL
Music in Place of Medication

As I made rounds the hospital, a nurse referred me to one of her patients. This was the first time I had been in contact with this nurse, but she seemed to know exactly what kind of patients benefit the most from music therapy. She told me the patient uncharacteristically, suddenly began crying.

When I visited the patient, she shook and sobbed with a tissue in her hand. I asked about her tears. She explained she was upset for waiting for so many years to get hip surgery. That she could have gotten surgery when she was in her twenties, but instead waited until she was eighty-three years old. She explained a summary of her life history; because she was so verbose, I asked if she wanted to write a song. We sang through "Home on the Range," and she filled in the blanks creating the following song:

"Home" (To the tune of "Home on the Range")
Oh, give me a home,
Where my son plays trombone,
But he's quiet most of the time!
Well, he married Fay.
She taught the 5th grade,
And she bakes cookies real well

Home, home in my town!
Where all the grandchildren stay.
Where they like their fish,
But not in a dish,
And they'll be here for three more days!

The nurse entered the room during the songwriting experience and asked the patient if she wanted a pain pill. The patient said, "Oh no, honey. I feel much better since I'm doing music!" The patient performed the song, to my guitar accompaniment, for two nurses passing by in the hallway. At the end of the treatment, the patient described her pain and anxiety as "zero."

The patient's assigned nurse had been on lunch break during the music therapy treatment. She was concerned about why her patient was upset prior to the session. I explained the happenings of the music therapy session. We concluded that the patient was probably feeling lonely because her roommate was recently discharged. Perhaps her loneliness, combined with stress from surgery, triggered anxiety and sadness. Working with both nurses was such a good, collaborative experience. Their knowledge of the benefits of music therapy impressed me. I feel so fortunate to be able to work with such an open-minded and educated medical staff.

A THOUGHTLESS INTERRUPTION
Working with Difficult Professionals

The patient was in bed, the lights were off, and she looked tired. She said she had pain in her back, rating it at a seven out of ten. She asked me to play music to help her sleep. I began a relaxing progression and prompted a deep breathing exercise. But a few minutes into the session, a nurse loudly entered the room, turned the lights on, spoke to the patient, and then drew some blood. I played my guitar throughout all of this... and held my tongue.

The nurse paid no attention to me, nor did she make any attempt to be quiet or consider the patient's environment. I felt that she was being rude. It would have been easy for her to say, "Sorry to interrupt. This will just take a minute." Luckily, I was playing relaxing music, which kept me calm enough to consider the situation instead of making a discourteous comment to the nurse. I knew that the nurse had a job to do, but so did I.

I remained silent while the nurse went about her business. The relaxation intervention picked up where I had left off, ad-libbing some lines regarding the interruption.

When I finished, the patient was asleep. What I learned is that I need to put the "Do Not Disturb – Music Therapy in Progress" sign on the door. I'm sure that this nurse will not be the last impolite person that I encounter on the job. I just need to remain calm and professional.

A JOINT EFFORT
Co-Treating with Physical Therapy

The physical therapist saw me and asked if I was coming to their patient's room for music therapy services. She explained that she was about to work with the patient, and I offered to provide music to reinforce goals. She agreed and explained that the patient had been experiencing hallucinations throughout the day. They wanted to keep him focused on reality while working on standing and balance skills.

I greeted the patient, and he returned the greeting with a smile. He stated he was glad I was there to see him. Despite the smile, his brow was furrowed. Conversations with his wife suggested it was due to frustration with being in the hospital and his inability to transfer himself from bed to chair. As the physical therapist began, I used neurological music therapy skills to provide complementary music for the tasks the patient was attempting: dynamic balance, weight shifting, deep breathing, and standing. Song selections included those requested by the patient.

The patient became distressed when trying to stand due to his tendency to fall backward and the weakness of his leg muscles. As a result, his breathing became rapid and I could see his blood pressure rising on the vital signs monitor.

I switched to a minor accompaniment pattern, humming and improvising a melody. The physical therapist encouraged the patient to focus on the music and his breathing; his blood pressure soon returned to regulated levels. I continued the musical relaxation as the physical therapist returned the patient to his bed. As we prepared to leave, the patient was visibly less distressed. He commented that the music sounded like a "turtledove" and confirmed that he enjoyed it.

When I said goodbye, he reached out his hand and held it for a moment to indicate his appreciation. Boldness pays off. I was not expecting to have an opportunity to work with a physical therapist, but I saw the opportunity and seized it. I learn a lot each time I co-treat and observe physical and occupational therapists working with patients.

A PROFESSIONAL CHORUS
Procedural Support with Music

Halfway through the first song with a patient, a nurse entered the room pushing a dialysis machine. "Great," I thought, "Just when it was looking like a great intervention, we get interrupted."

This kind of thing seems to happen far too frequently to me. I can't really complain since the primary purpose of a hospital stay is physiological treatment; music therapy serves a more auxiliary function. However, this visit seemed to have real potential. The patient was already singing and dancing in bed on the first song. Oh well, on to the next room.

Out of the depths of my mind, I heard my supervisor's voice challenging me to see how I could continue to facilitate a positive music experience under these circumstances. As I finished the first song, I turned to the nurse, offered a welcome, and stated that we were making music. Seeming to pick up on my underlying intention, the nurse exclaimed, "Well, don't stop on account of me!"

> **LESSONS LEARNED**
>
> *"Having the courage to create an opportunity for a successful music intervention can really pay off."*

Without missing a beat, the patient requested a song and soon all three of us were singing. Another nurse walked in the room and began prepping the patient for dialysis. Without hesitating, he joined us as we belted out the final chorus. At the close of the song, we laughed and cheered to accompany the dialysis prep work. The patient requested one more song before they turned the dialysis machine on, and I gladly obliged. Afterward, we all thanked each other for participating and traded smiles. I left the room in a positive mood; certain that everyone else involved had also received a boost.

SWEET APPRECIATION
Staff Involvement

My patient sat at his table as I asked how he was doing that day. He faintly responded, "Just fine." Hearing him tell me how he was doing was great, since I had previously only heard him speak once or twice.

The session was full of enthusiasm. The patient's nurse joined by singing and playing rhythm instruments. Soon, two more nurses came from down the hall. They had heard the music and wanted to be a part of it. Suddenly, the three nurses were dancing in front of the patient, playing instruments, and singing wildly. One more nurse came in the room. Before I knew it, I was in the middle of a show choir of nurses, singing, dancing, and waving rhythm instruments everywhere.

The nurses that joined our group left after a while, and the first nurse and I continued. The patient began to get sleepy, but he was still aware of the music, as I noticed him tapping his hand on the table. I decided that a slower song might be more appropriate to assist him in resting. I sang "What a Wonderful World."

I said goodbye and took his hand to shake it. He took my hand and kissed it; a sweet gesture from a sweet man.

I learned how important music might be for medical staff. Musical involvement between staff and patients can enhance their relationships and improve team morale. This session was fun for everyone.

Chapter 8: Questions for Growth

1. At the beginning of this chapter, Charles Darwin is quoted as follows: "In the long history of humankind, those who learned to collaborate and improvise most effectively have prevailed." Why has the author chosen this quote?

2. The therapist in the first excerpt of this chapter made a decision to see the patient who was obviously in pain and needed her attention immediately while she was present. Did she make the right decision to see this patient and miss her scheduled appointment with another patient? If so, how does she explain to the patient why she missed her appointment?

3. In the medical setting, working with others is inevitable. How might a therapist effectively build community between themselves and nurses or staff on the floors? How can they accomplish this with music?

4. What kind of stress-buster and/or group-building activity would you recommend for staff at a facility and what are some things that we can learn from the nursing staff in hospitals?

5. What is an experience you have had with a difficult professional? How did you carry through the session?

6. Why must music therapists always be in communication with the interdisciplinary team? List five important reasons.

7. Notice the subtext in "A Sparkling Referral: Music in Place of Medication." Have you noticed a shift in your medical community? Are people mostly inclined to pharmacological treatment, or are they shifting towards alternative medicine?

Chapter 9 · It's Not You, It's Me

"Sure I am this day we are masters of our
fate, that the task which has been set
before us is not above our strength; that its
pangs and toils are not beyond our
endurance. As long as we have faith in our
cause and an unconquerable will to win,
victory will not be denied us."

—Winston Churchill

A Successful Session
Not Giving Up After an Initial Decline

After a few declines, I was a bit frustrated but still determined to see patients. I saw that a patient referred for social interaction had responded well to music therapy the previous day.

The patient was lying in bed with his wife and daughter by his side. He looked tired but greeted me with a wave. He said that he enjoyed music therapy, but he was having a rough day and did not have the energy for a session. His daughter looked at me and said that he was having trouble sleeping; he tossed and turned a lot because of his pain.

I said I would gladly come back another time, but I mentioned that music therapy is also geared towards facilitating relaxation to help patients sleep. She looked puzzled, so I began to fingerpick Pachelbel's Canon in C.

After a few chord changes, the patient had closed his eyes and his body visibly relaxed. He was on his way to dreamland. I played for about five minutes; when I was sure that he was asleep I slowly faded out the music.

His daughter and wife both mouthed "Thank You" to me as I quietly exited the room.

> ❧ LESSONS LEARNED ❧
>
> *"It is our responsibility as therapists to be open to all of the possibilities for a session. Even when people initially refuse, they can still benefit."*

Even though people may have received music therapy, they may not know the extent of its capabilities. Music therapists use music in association with the isoprinciple to meet clients where they are physically, mentally, and emotionally.

IT DEPENDS

Dealing with a Difficult Client

I could tell that this man was going to be a challenge from our initial conversation. I asked him how prominent his pain was, and he said, "Depends." I then said, "It depends on what?" He replied, "Well, it depends. Are you asking about pain in my foot or where?"

I then explained that I wanted to know his general level of pain, hoping this was easier for him to understand. The only response he gave me was "it depends," so I decided to move on and ask him about his music preferences.

I asked what type of music he enjoyed, he replied, "It depends." Instead of trying to explore this explanation, I said, "Yes, I guess what we like to listen to depends on our mood that day." I took out a songbook and gave him a choice between two songs. He wasn't able to make a choice, so I started singing "Fly Me to the Moon." He engaged in eye contact and active listening while I sang. After I finished, I asked him if he liked any specific artists, and he replied, "I don't see any potential for this music because the music I listen to is on a program." I asked what kind of music was featured on the program, but he did not answer. I suggested we try one last song. I sang through the first stanza and continued to play the chords. I asked if he recognized this song. He said, "Yes, but like I said, I don't really see any potential for this music because the music I listen to is on a program." I finally found out that he listened to a television program every day at three o'clock. I felt there was nothing else I could do, so I apologized that I could not offer any music that he liked. I asked if he was planning to watch his television program that day, and without fail, he responded, "It depends." I then told him it was nice to meet him and packed up my stuff to leave.

This difficult session discouraged and frustrated me. I am not sure what I could have done differently. Maybe I just didn't click with this patient.

THE COLD SHOULDER
Understanding The Patient Perspective

When I arrived at the hospital, a nurse referred a patient to me who would love to hear some music. I entered the room and saw the patient sitting up in bed, alert, with the television on and a magazine on her table.

I introduced myself and mentioned that her nurse had asked me to come see her. I asked her about her pain and anxiety level, which she rated at a ten and nine, respectively. I nodded to show that I heard and understood what she said and was about to open my mouth again to explain how we could use music to help with her pain and anxiety. Instead, she said sharply, "You know what, I don't have time for this. I'm supposed to get my pain pill now."

Again, I nodded and began to explain that after she got her pill, we could use music and relaxation techniques to help bridge the gap until the medicine took effect. "Did my nurse really send you?" she demanded. I repeated that she had.

The patient said she wanted to call her nurse and picked up her call button. When the front desk answered, she asked for her nurse to come to her room "right now." She then turned back to me, saying in a loud, irritated tone, "Look, I'm not trying to be rude, but I don't have time for this." I managed to pull an informational card from the cart to hand to her before retreating. I left the room feeling quite on edge and no longer sympathetic about her pain. This was the harshest decline I have ever received. I barely had a chance to offer services before this woman kicked me out of her room. I was surprised by how quickly I responded to her behavior personally, becoming increasingly angry. Reflecting on this situation after reading the patient's chart in more detail, I saw that psychiatric issues and drug-seeking behaviors were an issue. I was indeed invading this patient's space at a sensitive time. I always try to remember that declines of services are not because I am a bad therapist.

NEGATIVE NANCY
It's the Roommate

When I entered my patient's room, I first saw a smiling, gray-haired woman. As we spoke, she appeared to have severe dementia as evidenced by her inability to answer simple questions and the presence of a baby doll in her arms. The nurse entered and confirmed my suspicions.

The nurse said that the patient would enjoy music therapy and she had been singing, "Jesus Loves Me" all morning to herself. When I mentioned the song and asked the patient to sing it, she immediately began in a loud and self-assured voice, missing some of the words, but hitting every note. When I began to sing with her, a huge smile spread across her face and her eyes seemed to say, "No one has ever done that before." After a short song, I was ready to bring in the songbooks and the guitar, but I wanted to ask her roommate if it was alright with her to do some music.

I wasn't prepared for what happened next. The patient's younger roommate was already agitated, stomping around her side of the room, yelling, "No, it's not alright, but you already woke me up and I was just about to fall asleep!"

I quickly apologized and told her that the music therapy team never begins a session without the neighbor's permission and I could always come back at a better time. "No! No! No!" the woman yelled. "You need to be more considerate. What's wrong with you? I can't believe this!"

Thankfully at that moment, the nurse entered and the woman rushed out of the room. "She's just crabby," the nurse said. "And besides, her roommate needs music therapy." I explained to the nurse that I did not want to force the patient to leave the room on account of music therapy. But, the nurse insisted I continue with my patient and that her neighbor could find a place to sit for five minutes. I got my guitar, regained my composure and approached my patient again, who did not seem to be affected by the incident. While we were singing, another nurse entered the room and was shocked to see the patient's large smile. "Wow," she said, "she's really responding to this. I haven't seen her this happy since she's been here. We usually can't even get a smile."

I left a little shaken, but with a lesson learned. I must always check to see if the second patient in a room is sleeping before approaching the first. Most of the time, a neighbor who is sleeping is not bothered by the music; however, some patients may be put off by it. I think I handled the situation as best I could. I will be prepared for the patients who do not want my services in the future.

A NEW APPROACH
Trying a New Way to Get in the Door

On my first time seeing patients without supervision, everything was going well. When I realized my next referral was a client who had declined music therapy services several times in the past month, I grew nervous. I knew that none of the interns had been able to get into her room to provide treatment. I made up my mind that I would do my best to turn her "no" into a "yes."

I prepared myself and planned what I was going to say to make her feel comfortable enough to agree to treatment. I took a deep breath and entered the room. The patient was lying in bed and her husband sat at her bedside.

I told her that I saw from her charts that she has been in the hospital for quite some time. She said, "That's an understatement." I told her I understood that it must be challenging for her and asked her if she had any pain. She reported her pain at eight out of ten scale. I asked if she would mind if I provided relaxing music to see if it helped with the pain and gave her the option to hear just one or two songs. She said, "I guess one song would be fine."

The patient chose a song that she said she used to sing with her father. As I was playing, the patient sang along, saying the song brought back great memories. I asked the couple if they had any songs that were special to them as a couple. The husband said they have several but named one in particular, "Better Together" by Jack Johnson. I was unfamiliar with the song, but he brought it up on his phone and began to play it.

Within the first thirty seconds of the song, both the patient and her husband began to cry. He stood up and hugged her, cheek to cheek. In the background, the lyrics expressed how life is hard and can be deceiving, but everything is "better when we're together." The patient whispered, "I love you," and her husband returned the words.

When the song ended, I commented on how beautiful the song was and that they are both lucky to have each other during these hard times. They shared that throughout their thirty years of marriage, they never gave up in hard times, and always encouraged each other to get through things together. I asked the patient at the end of the session about her pain level. She reported that it felt a little less intense and that the music was "a good diversion" from the pain. I was pleased to hear that. I said goodbye to the couple and walked out of the room thinking, "That was awesome."

LESSONS LEARNED

"Even the most unlikely patient can be an excellent candidate for music therapy."

One can never know when a patient might finally say 'yes' to music therapy, even though they have declined several times in the past. Sometimes all it takes is a different approach.

GET OUT OF MY ROOM
Honoring a Patient's Request

The hospital staff had a mixture of strained and jovial attitudes on this particular day. I discreetly moved through the crowded nurses' station, stealthily seeking out another referral.

The charge nurse kindly provided me with a few patients. She spoke of one but said, "She may throw you out of the room. She's really confused and difficult." I noted the friendly warning and prepared my mind for the imminent challenge. I was curious to see how long I could engage this woman in a musical intervention.

As I entered the room, I was greeted graciously by the patient and welcomed to her bedside for "a song or two." I had barely finished positioning my guitar when the patient began a high-pitched wail: "Please get me out of here! They won't let me go!" Her nurse was quick to assure her that she would leave the instant she was able to walk. The patient started to pry at the foam cast on her leg, which prompted an immediate countered response from the nurse.

What an excellent time for a song. I opened my songbook and allowed the music to do its job. The patient stopped crying and looked at me as I sang. She blinked a few times, sat back in her bed, and shifted her gaze to the other end of the room. She did not have any memories connected with "America the Beautiful," but she said she wished I would just tell 'those people' (the staff) to let her go. The nurses shot me apologetic glances and encouraged the patient to pay attention to the music.

Somehow, I was able to sing four songs, engage the patient in reminiscence about her dog, and write a parody about how much she missed her home. I sang with abandon, doing my best to support the nurse's desire for her to eat some gelatin and to distract her from painful needle pokes. The last event proved too much for the patient, and she asked me to leave.

That I could do. I smiled and wished her well in her recovery. The patient's frown disappeared as she gazed back at me, mystified by the results of her request, and thanked me for visiting. Finally, she was able to tell someone else what to do. I chuckled on my way out; so this is what it's like to be thrown out of a room!

Carrying a spirit of joy into each session is important. We can't take everything seriously, especially when asked to leave. A patient's choices should be honored because the decision to have music therapy may be one of the only things they can control during their hospital stay.

FINDING AN "IN"
Incorporating Music in New Ways

I had visited this patient several times since his admittance to the hospital, but rarely found him alert and available for a session. I entered the room and he greeted me warmly, telling me that he remembered me stopping by previously. We talked about his treatment; the patient told me that he was not doing well. When asked if he would like music therapy, he declined, but continued discussing various topics with me.

The patient eventually discussed his musical preferences and knowing that he was a guitar player, I stated that his life right now sounded like a blues song. He smiled and told me that if I played it, he would sing it. I began to play a blues progression. He did not sing the blues, but he did begin speaking in rhythm with the music. We continued speaking the blues for quite some time. He thanked me and said he would enjoy it if I came again to do some more blues.

✄ LESSONS LEARNED ✄

"Never give up. Never, never, never, never."

When he initially declined services, I began looking for a way to excuse myself from the room so I could move on to the next patient. He kept talking and talking, and I soon realized that I should not be looking for a way out of the room, rather a way to use music in the room to help the patient express himself.

I found that opportunity when he told me he used to play the blues. All it took was taking a breath, pulling out my guitar, and playing a simple chord progression to engage this patient in a successful intervention. I learned that with persistence comes success.

CHAPTER 9: QUESTIONS FOR GROWTH

1. In one way or another, most of the stories in this chapter tell of declines, or negative responses to music therapy. If a patient declines a session in a medical setting with a certain reason (wants to sleep, no energy, etc.), what are some ways you may be able to extend other services to them? What's an experience you've had with declines? What lesson did you learn, if any, from it?

2. Suppose a potential patient's roommate gets upset over your services, claims they are a distraction, and refuses to leave the room. There are no available nurses around the room. How would you handle the situation?

3. As said in this chapter, "With persistence comes success." When is being persistent for an approval for music therapy rather than a decline from a patient inappropriate?

4. In this chapter we have read of a therapist who honored a patients request in leaving the room during therapy services with little to no rebuttal towards the patients request. Why was this the right thing to do?

5. Dealing with declines can be hard, especially when a client is rude about it. Why is it important to do follow-ups with clients in a hospital setting even if they give a rude decline one day?

6. In the excerpt, "It Depends" from this chapter, what might the therapist have done differently to be more successful with the client and the success of the session?

Chapter 10 - I'm Not With the Band!

*"A beautiful sunset that was mistaken for
a dawn."*

—Claude Debussy

Doctor's Orders
Conceived as "Unimportant"

The first time I walked into the patient's room, a CNA was sitting in a chair in the room reading a book in a contact precaution gown. The patient was lying in bed, eyes closed, snoring loudly. The CNA told me, "He just sleeps all day, but we have him restrained because he is disoriented when he wakes up."

I began to play slow arpeggios in an effort to match his breathing, which proved to be difficult, because it was quite sporadic. After a few minutes, his breathing was close enough to a steady rhythm that I decided to take the lead and see if he'd follow. Thirty minutes into the session, I sang "Amazing Grace" – things got interesting. Halfway through the song, the patient grimaced, opened his eyes, looked up at the wall, and then over to me. He continued to snore, but with his eyes wide open. For the next thirty minutes, he remained this way. The amazed CNA said, "This is the longest he's stayed awake yet!"

When I got back to the office, I found three more referrals. One confused me; it was from the same doctor to see the same patient again. I thought, "This must be a typo," and started to write this on the referral, when I thought to myself, "Maybe it's a second referral." To confirm my suspicions, I listened to the phone message and discovered a request to see the patient again.

When I returned, the excited nurse said the doctor was so happy with the result the day before that he wanted music therapy again the next day. This time, the patient's wife was in the room. He was once again snoring loudly with his eyes shut. She thanked me for what I did during the previous session. I asked if she had any personal requests and she listed some music that her husband loved. Today, I increased my vocal volume since it was clear that they wanted me to wake him again.

Once again, when I sang "Amazing Grace," the patient grimaced and opened his eyes again. His wife exclaimed, "That's the first time I've seen those beautiful blue eyes all day!" I continued to play the requested songs (patriotic marches). The nurse for the patient next door asked us to shut the door; moments later, she returned and said the patient in the next room was agitated because he could still hear me through the wall. She asked me to stop the "entertainment" all together.

When I told my patient's nurse what happened, she was immediately upset. The neighbor was apparently discharging to go home the next day. The nurse felt that my patient's needs were more important. I felt apologetic for upsetting a patient; it was unfortunate to leave such a successful session on those circumstances.

The music was not for entertainment; it was a clinical treatment referred twice by a doctor. Yet, I immediately fell into apologies. Thinking back on it, while I need to respect others' space and take it down a notch if I'm too loud, they also need to respect what I am doing. Next time, I will inform the nurse I will lower my volume but continue treating a patient per the doctor's request. If the nurse wishes to escalate the issue, I will refer her to the doctor.

TRUST ME
The Proof is in the Research

I was in the elevator on my way up when a woman said to me, "Oh, how nice. Music therapy!" She asked me some questions about who we see. I knew we were going to the same floor, so I asked if she had any referrals. She told me about her mom and gave me the room number, and I assured her I would be there soon.

The first time I passed the room, the doctor was talking with the family and it seemed like the patient was still having some pain. I finished up with other patients and then went back to the room. The patient's daughter was sitting beside her mother and recognized me. She introduced me to the patient and told me that her mother used to play and teach piano. The patient was frail, very sweet, and she readily welcomed me to her bedside. I offered to play some familiar tunes to sing.

The patient's daughter leaned in and said, "Maybe not. She has dementia, she won't remember them." I told her she'd be surprised and continued on, though the daughter seemed skeptical. Sure enough, once I began with some tunes from the patient's teenage years, she was singing nearly every word along with me. As we were singing, the daughter stepped away and began talking to her husband and said, "She said I'd be surprised."

After working with the patient for about fifteen minutes, I talked to the daughter and mentioned the music therapy research that's been done with Alzheimer's and dementia diagnoses. She was impressed with the research and with the way her mother had responded.

We are constant educators. Showing the family how music can work and back it up with the research was interesting. By her response, I think the daughter was surprised by seeing her mother sing. This experience gives her a positive and more understanding attitude towards music therapy.

A PRIVATE PERFORMANCE
Riding the Line Between Music Therapist and Performer

I was seeing a follow-up patient, when the husband of the patient in the next room came to the door and asked if I would come see his wife next. When I entered the room, bringing along my violin, guitar, ukulele, and music books, the patient immediately smiled. She told me that she had studied musicology and she enjoyed folk and classical music the most. I was thankful to have my violin, but I contemplated how to make this visit about music therapy and not a performance.

I invited the patient to close her eyes and let the music do for her whatever she needed at that moment. I began with a folk tune on violin and watched as the patient smiled, closed her eyes at times, and relaxed. Her husband commented that the music brought tears to his eyes, which gave me the opportunity to point out how music can affect our emotions and mood.

After the folk piece, the patient requested some classical music. I played a short portion of a Bach piece on violin. During this part of the session, I began to feel more like a performer rather than a therapist. I know that the music was therapeutic for the patient because I could see her affect change and she said that the music had improved her mood. The patient shared with me that she sang in a church choir, so I offered to finish the session with a hymn on guitar. We finished the session by singing together; the patient even added some harmony. The patient and her husband were grateful for the music - both said that it brightened their day.

I feel like more of a therapist when I'm playing guitar with vocal accompaniment. As soon as I pick up my violin, I have trouble staying in the mindset of a therapist, partly because I sense that other people view me as a performer when they hear and see the instrument. I know I am capable of using the violin therapeutically, but others may not recognize this function as readily.

Educating patients, families, and staff about our role as therapists is critical. Pointing out my observations about the effect of the music on the patient's body or mood puts me more into the therapist role rather than a performer.

THE CONCERT HALL
Giving Clients What They Need

I had seen this patient the previous week. She was a nice, personable, and friendly woman. Her daughter was with her on this occasion.

We chatted a bit about our last visit and about her granddaughter. After I played two songs, the patient and her daughter clapped and smiled, as though I had given a concert. I wanted somehow to give the patient more than 'just a concert,' but she was not in pain, not in poor spirits, and not lonely or depressed.

I realized that this "concert" was probably just what she needed at that moment. I should not underestimate the fact that our mere presence and the music can be therapeutic for some clients. If a "concert" is what is going to benefit the client the most - if that's what is called for, then that's what I'll do.

CHAPTER 10: QUESTIONS FOR GROWTH

1. In the first excerpt, the therapist is confronted with a dilemma of whether or not she did the right thing by ending a successfully progressing session at the request of the nurse of the patient next door. Review the excerpt and discuss what would be the most appropriate course of action.

2. In "A Private Performance," the therapist felt like a performer due to the difference in instruments being used. Was she correct in her understanding of her role? Does an instrument make the difference in your role as a therapist versus a performer?

3. What are some ways you can redirect staff or family when they refer to music therapy as entertainment? How can you educate them?

4. List five differences and similarities between a music therapist and a performer.

5. How do you differentiate between a performance and a music therapy session when the only intervention accomplished by the patient it active listening?

Chapter 11 - Jaw-Dropping: Those Exceptional Moments

*"I love to hear a choir. I love the humanity
to see the faces of real people devoting
themselves to a piece of music. I like the
teamwork. It makes me feel optimistic
about the human race when I see them
cooperating like that."*

–Paul McCartney

Bringing Back a Memory

A Patient with Memory Loss

The patient sat in a chair near the window; illuminated by the sunshine in the relative darkness of his room. He had suffered a stroke and now found difficulty with memory and reading. During our previous session, he had been trying to recall a favorite song of his.

Today, he seemed excited because he had remembered one line from the song and sang it for us: "Even though we ain't got money." During the rest of the session, we read some song titles to the patient; he chose a few and asked us to pick some. The patient closed his eyes or looked out the window and thanked us after each song was finished. He said it had been a bad night, but listening to the music helped him not to think about it.

Once or twice, the patient began to cry, saying that it was "so frustrating" not to be able to remember the words to songs he used to know. We responded with active listening and validated his feelings. At the close of the session, I told him I would return with the song he requested.

The next time I saw the patient, he was waiting to be discharged. His spirits seemed much higher, and he was glad to hear I found the song: "Danny's Song" by Kenny Loggins. He seemed so relieved to know the name of the song and the artist, saying, "I never would have remembered that. Thank you so much." As I played, he laid his head back and closed his eyes. He began to cry softly and sometimes sang the lines he remembered. When I finished, he thanked me again, saying, "I used to sing that song to my little girl, who I lost to cancer."

He talked about the recent events in his life since the stroke. "After being so lucky all my life, to never have any physical limitations," he said, "now I can barely read. I just have to sit here and watch TV. I can't remember the things that were important to me - the details. I looked at myself in the mirror the other day and barely recognized myself. Sometimes I just sit and feel so sorry for myself. But when you are here, and even just seeing you, it makes everything better." I expressed how happy I was that music therapy had helped him so much. After the session was over, I left him with a copy of the song, so he could remember the title.

This was definitely one of those, "Yes, this is why I'm doing this" moments. It was also one of those 'right place at the right time' moments. The fact that I knew this random song from the 1970s he had requested empowered me; not many people my age know that song. I was able to find it, learn it, and help give the patient back a part of his memory that he was struggling to recover. This experience showed me, once again, the unique power of music therapy and helped renew my sense of purpose.

MOVING THROUGH EMOTIONS
Prepping a Patient for Physical Therapy

When I entered a referred patient's room, she was lying in bed watching television with a pouty look on her face. I asked her how she felt, and she replied sadly, "OK, I guess." She said that her pain was up to ten (out of ten scale). She asked what kind of music I play, and I gave her some choices. We sang and played Willie Nelson's song, "Crazy."

After the song, the physical therapist arrived. This arrival proved to be an emotional trigger for the patient as she started ranting and raving about her pain. Their conversation ended in friendly sarcasm, and he left for a few minutes.

When he left, she was fired up about the day's events, her face flushed, her brow furrowed, and her hands shaking in anger. I started playing the blues loudly and repeating her words and interjecting. She immediately chimed in with melodious statements: "I'm always being moved from here to there!" "This is so ridiculous!" "I don't have the strength to walk!" "I'll hardly make it out the door!" "I don't want to do it!" "I just got here!" "How can he expect me to do this?" We continued until her words gradually became calmer and slower.

Finally, she let out a big sigh and a chuckle. I asked her why she had to do physical therapy, and from there, the "Benefits of Physical Therapy Improvised Blues" was born. She sang, "It's good to get the blood going," "It's good for my muscle strength," "It helps me get better." The physical therapist returned in the middle of this song, and he chimed in with more benefit statements: "It helps to maintain your strength and motor movement ability," and "It's good for circulation."

As we were packing up and making our way to the door, the physical therapist asked her how she was feeling after music therapy. She replied in a humorous tone, "Well, I'm feeling better than I was before." She thanked us in the end and self-reported her pain as an eight.

This experience seemed so cathartic. The patient was gathered, contained, and then released through the music. Music was the vehicle for self-expression and, in the end, provided resolution. I also believe that the songwriting experience motivated her, because later in the day she walked all the way down the hall, contrary to her previous prediction.

WARMING THE SOUL
A Woman with Post-Birth Complications

When the social worker made this referral, she explained that the patient had recently given birth to twins. Now she was in the hospital with complications and was experiencing postpartum depression. I expected to focus on comfort support, diversion, and providing an opportunity for emotional expression. I knew my plans would have to change as soon as I entered her room. Her fever had spiked and she was experiencing severe chills causing uncontrollable shaking and difficulty breathing. I asked if she would be interested in some music and relaxation exercises. She agreed and when I entered, she said, "Oh, you mean live music. I thought you had recordings."

As the nurse layered on more blankets, tightly wrapped up the patient, and added medication to her IV, I began to play the guitar in a fast, yet steady picking pattern. The patient said that if she could get her breathing under control, the chills usually subsided. I led her in a deep breathing exercise; I gradually decreased the tempo as her breathing became more even and the chills became less visibly noticeable. I continued to play softly as the patient practiced deep breathing.

Several minutes later, she opened her eyes again saying, 'Thank you. That really helped." Her roommate commented that the music had put her to sleep. The patient asked if I knew Pachelbel's "Canon in D." I told her, "Yes," and encouraged her to close her eyes again as I played it on violin. She thanked me for helping her get her breathing under control and said she was feeling much better.

As I was leaving, the nurse stopped me to express her appreciation. She said the music seemed to ease the patient's symptoms and she was glad I'd provided services.

TAKING AWAY THE FEAR
Supporting a Child through Chemotherapy

I was working in pediatrics when I decided to see a young girl diagnosed with cancer and about to begin chemotherapy treatments. She was fearful and anxious as several nurses gathered around her to set up IVs and tubes for chemotherapy. The patient began crying when she saw the nurses setting up the treatment. Her mother immediately asked us to stay. I asked her what songs she liked and we began singing several of her favorites, attempting to distract her from her fear and anxiety.

At first, the patient rarely participated; she briefly glanced at me and then stared at the ground. Soon, she increased the duration of eye contact. She smiled, reached for and then played an egg shaker to "Twist and Shout" and "Egg Shakin' Blues." During this time, nurses discreetly finished setting up and began the chemotherapy treatment while the patient remained distracted. Throughout the music-making experience, her mother and several nurses smiled and provided appreciative, thankful glances that I was in the room with them.

Several minutes after the chemotherapy treatment began, the patient started coughing and placed her hands over her stomach. Her face drained of color and she began sweating. She immediately leaned over in her chair and cried in pain. She complained that her stomach hurt. Her mother began crying as well, and she called for a nurse. I stepped back, and quickly began playing calm lullabies on the guitar and humming. As the nurse moved the patient to her bed, I turned down the lights and instructed her to close her eyes as I continued humming and playing. Within a few minutes, she was sound asleep, a slight smile on her face.

I witnessed the powerful effects of music therapy that day, specifically the benefits of music therapy in providing procedural support, increasing relaxation, and relieving pain. This session reaffirmed why I want to be a music therapist, why I believe music therapy works, and why music therapy needs to be a part of pediatric care.

DANCE OF A LIFETIME
Giving the Patient What They Always Needed

On our first visit to the patient's room, my co-therapist and I found him to be a wonderfully positive man with an inspiring outlook on life. We learned that he was a helpful, caring individual and that he loved to go dancing with his wife. Unfortunately, many years had passed since they were able to go because she was also very ill and had lost the ability to move around by herself. Now with his illness, he could only express the desire to dance again. Since we had such a good session, I decided to follow-up with him when I was on the floor by myself.

Once again, he was in a bright and cheery mood. He requested many songs and happily sang and played along with me. He especially enjoyed a blues song we improvised with some sayings he had posted on his wall. After a bit of singing and storytelling, he again spoke of his desire to dance. I invited him to do so by telling him that I have always wanted to go dancing but that my significant other has two left feet.

He proceeded to say, "But it's so easy! I could show you some things to show him." He said we did not have enough room in his hospital room, so we proceeded to the activity room at the end of the hall. Once there, we began to dance. Nurses and visitors came into the room to watch him, and they all applauded at the end of our dance. I made sure to not dance for too long because of his weakened state, but it was wonderful for both of us.

As we walked back to his room, I thanked him for showing me how to dance. He smiled from ear to ear and thanked me for a wonderful experience. He said he had never guessed that the hospital would be the place where he got to dance again. It meant so much to him. I was pleased that I had the chance to fulfill a wish for this man and provide him with a dance partner. He stated that our dance had made his week, and I felt the same way.

STAND BY ME
Helping a Woman Relax Before Surgery

I had introduced myself to a patient the day before, and she said she was excited for music. She said her husband played many instruments and he would love it too. I started the session with a music and relaxation exercise. She opened her eyes at the end of it and smiled. I asked her if she did deep breathing on her own and she replied, "Yes, but the music really helps."

She then chose some songs for us to sing. Her husband told us that she used to sing, that her voice was as sweet as a bird. "I wish you'd sing more," he told her. She said it had been years and she could not sing well anymore. The patient laid back and listened to a few more songs with a smile; she hummed along with the melody from time to time. The last song "You've Got a Friend" was one she and her husband had sung together at their wedding thirty-two years ago. I began singing it, and soon, both of them joined me quietly. By the end of it, I faded my voice out so it was just the two of them. Their beautiful duet moved me almost to tears.

"This is great. It would be nice to have you come all the way down to my surgery," the patient said.

"I might be able to do that," I said. "I'll talk to your nurse and let you know."

As I left the room, I wondered how it would work to go all the way down to surgery with her. I'd never done it before, but anything is possible. Her nurse said to give it a shot, so I did.

I waited until the staff came to take the patient down. As they rolled her down the hallway to the elevator, I began singing softly. The patient closed her eyes and sang along with me. On our way, an employee passed by us and looked perplexed, as if she couldn't believe what she saw. I continued to sing as we waited for the elevator and got onto it. We continued on the elevator ride and transitioned to a quiet hum. The patient's eyes were closed, and she had a smile on her face. We exited the elevator as if we were in our own bubble. When we arrived, she thanked me and said she'd be fine from there. I felt an incredible energy from her.

An Emotional Moment
A Patient's Powerful Support System

I found myself standing at the foot of a patient's bed surrounded by two other music therapists and five of the patient's friends. We were all singing, "When the night has come, and the land is dark, and the moon is the only light we'll see..."

I began to think of the significance of the lyrics. Five friends were singing to support their friend who was going to have surgery the next day. We continued to sing, "No, I won't be afraid, just as long as you stand, stand by me." The patient and I made eye contact, and we smiled at each other. I tried to understand what the look in her eyes meant. I wondered what was going through her mind and what she was feeling. She seemed like a child hiding under the covers, scared and wanting the situation to disappear, but putting on a brave face. "Oh, I won't cry, no I won't shed a tear, just as long as you stand by me." Tears began to well in my eyes, and I couldn't continue to sing. I looked away from the client hoping

> ✖ LESSONS LEARNED ✖
>
> *"It is important to be aware of oneself and remember that even though we are therapists, we are human beings, too."*

that she wouldn't notice as I worked to pull myself together.

I found it extremely touching that this patient had so many people 'standing by her.' I thought of the importance of a support group to aid in her healing process. This session allowed me to feel firsthand the power that music can have on one's emotions. I also came face to face with my own emotions. This was the first time I struggled to keep my composure during a session.

A SURPRISE ENCOUNTER
Music Reaches an Unresponsive Patient

The case manager said that the patient had been non-responsive for three days. A note on the patient's tray table, in cursive and signed by her three children, said that they had come by to visit, but left since she was asleep. I decided to sing softly anyway.

I had difficulty determining whether or not she was asleep because her eyes were wide open. In fact, this juxtaposed presentation prompted me to check with the staff about her condition. The patient's heavy breathing, fixed gaze, hanging head, and non-responsiveness to music certainly indicated sleep, a partial coma, or some other sort of altered state of consciousness.

After two songs, the patient suddenly raised her head straight up, looked right at me, and with a smile spoke quietly, but with focus, "Thank you, thank you, thank you!" Even the nurse who happened to be in the room charting could not believe her eyes and ears.

Upon the patient's request, I continued to sing. The patient sang along with the more upbeat, even somewhat improvised version, of "He's Got the Whole World in His Hands," including a verse about her cat. This provided the patient with an opportunity to think, feel, and communicate about loved ones who were not present. She appeared exhausted, so I closed the session with a final song.

The patient repeated her gratitude and requested that I stop by anytime. The nurse once again expressed her amazement, and I left the room knowing that, despite the initial indication, music reached a soul and improved the quality of a woman's life that day.

CHAPTER 11: QUESTIONS FOR GROWTH

1. At the beginning of this chapter, Paul McCartney is quoted. Why has the author chosen this quote? How does this apply to the rest of the chapter?

2. Exceptional moments can fuel our success amongst times of trial in our profession. During those difficult times what are some activities that the therapist can do to remember those exceptional moments?

3. If you find yourself getting emotional in a session, what do you do? How would you handle the situation?

4. A therapist accompanied a patient to surgery in this chapter, and she said that she was given a lot of weird looks on her way. What do you think are some rational feelings that the therapist was feeling in that moment?

5. In one of the excerpts from this chapter, the therapist dances with a patient. Suppose the patient's physician approaches you later and tells you that the patient's illness requires the patient to reserve his strength and have limited movement. How do you respond?

6. Throughout this chapter, many "aha" moments are shared. Take a moment and share your three most memorable "aha's" so far.

7. Get into small groups and improvise on a blues melody about the events that are currently happening in the room.

Chapter 12 - The Butterfly: Spread Your Wings

"Just like the butterfly, I, too, will awaken in my own time."

–Deborah Chaskin

Gaining Confidence
Working with Medically Fragile Students

My supervisor had a presentation, so I was given the opportunity to run solo sessions at a school. This population was unfamiliar to me and we had not yet had consistent sessions with groups or individual sessions. I felt nervous about running the four individual and two group sessions that morning. Also, due to the hectic start of the school year for these children, some of their goals were not finalized in their IEPs, which caused me additional stress.

I began with my first one-on-one session of the day. I was surprised at how comfortable I was working with a 7-year-old fragile girl. I forgot about my nerves and had a great time with her and the rest of the students that I saw throughout the day. I was amazed that I was able to address each of the student's goals and objectives throughout our sessions together, and I was comfortable in doing so. Everything began to click and the work I was doing felt natural. I know it seems redundant, but it's true: I can trust myself. I can trust my clinical skills, but also felt that this experience of leading by myself brought me closer to these children and set the precedent for me to have more successful sessions in the future.

FINDING YOUR GROOVE

Reaching a Woman with a Long Medical History

For several months, I have been seeing a young woman in the midst of a long recovery process due to several surgeries pertaining to her gastrointestinal system. Many of our sessions focused on pain and anxiety management, as well as emotional expression.

More recently, I had been feeling disconnected from the patient. She declined music therapy several times, even though the social worker stated that the woman had been doing much better. After she had another surgery, she was open to music therapy again. We had a couple of pain management and relaxation sessions while she was in ICU. Still, I would walk away from the sessions not feeling like the therapy was as effective as possible. I decided to trust that our sessions would find their natural flow once more and that I would be able to provide the best therapy for her. This time, I was pleased to find that she had moved to the side of the ICU where more stable patients stay.

When I walked in, the patient smiled and seemed excited that I had come to see her. We sang a few of her favorite songs, including "The Rose." As I read the lyrics, I realized that it would be an excellent song for songwriting. After the song, I asked the patient what her idea of "love" is. I gradually led her into a songwriting experience, and she completed her own verse for the song. We sang it through, and she smiled widely.

"Some say love, it is trusting, loving until the end, some say love, it is everything. It is open, honest. Some say love, it's a songbird that is always there. I say love, it is magic, that binds your soul to me."

I told her that I would type the song lyrics for her, she was so pleased, I walked away from this session feeling that the "flow" was exactly what it needed to be and I felt that the therapeutic dynamic between the patient, the music, and myself was balanced. I was pleased to leave her with such a positive feeling.

TRYING SOMETHING NEW
Trusting Your Instinct During Sessions

My first group of the day was with patients who are in a day treatment program at a mental health center. For this group, I had prepared a songwriting exercise where the patients could not only write the lyrics of a song, but write the music as well. Because I had never done this type of exercise before, I was concerned that it would need some serious adjustments. I also somewhat expected the patients to lose interest and I would have to change direction and do something different.

We began the session with "The Friday Blues." I played a blues song on piano for each patient. I had written a song with the theme of "hope," and I had written two different versions of each line and each chord. This way, I could ask each patient to make a choice between two different phrases and later could ask the entire group for advice on the music. The song had three verses and a chorus, and almost every patient contributed by either choosing a phrase I had pre-written or by writing their own phrase for each verse and the chorus. When the song was complete, we sang through it several times.

What made this session significant was the overwhelmingly positive feedback I received. The patients seemed to enjoy the songwriting experience, too. One client wrote down the song with the lyrics and chords, and several others insisted on getting copies.

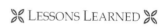

❈ LESSONS LEARNED ❈

"If you don't try, you'll never know how successful something could be."

Taking a risk and trusting in one's abilities as a therapist can be a milestone with great benefits.

PERFECT RECORD

Changing Your Strategy to Ensure Success

My first patient of the day was a woman with a gruff voice, sitting in bed, reading. I initially thought she would decline, but she hesitantly agreed to a music therapy session. The patient chose one song and then we started talking.

The more we talked, the more she started to open up and laugh. She explained the problem with her lungs and how she had to quit smoking. She was quite insightful about motivation, saying that in the past, people have nagged her and it didn't work. We discussed the difficulty of changing our thought patterns and the importance of focusing on a positive goal. The patient became fascinated with the Q-Chord. At the end of the session, the patient said, "This is a wonderful program. I am so glad you came today."

My next session was referred by the social worker because the patient was challenging for the staff. I had seen this patient three weeks prior and was left with the impression that the patient had difficulty remaining positive through their tough journey. The patient saw me enter her room and ended her phone call saying, "The music therapist is here, and I want to see her." She discussed her hospital stay and disclosed that she was not quite ready to go home, but was being discharged that day. She said, "Music helps to calm me down when I feel nauseous."

I convinced her to let me play some music for her. She said she loved the flute and also asked that I play guitar and sing. She said, "I have never had someone play music for me." She even smiled for the first time. As I was leaving, the patient said, "Thank you. You made my day. I don't feel nauseous now."

I had two additional sessions that day with similar outcomes: positive responses and no declines. I left that day feeling successful. Out of all the people I came in contact with, not one declined; it was my first time with a 100 percent success rate. First, I tried many different things, which I feel contributed to this successful day. My number one goal with patients was to learn about them and find a way to get them to open up. Second, I was more confident. I didn't allow myself to think before going into the patient's room or to undermine myself. I finally found my groove.

THE LEARNING CURVE
Sessions that Make You Think

When I entered the patient's room earlier in the day, she was getting dressed and prepped for her discharge. Her daughter said, "She won't be leaving for a while, so come back later. My mom loves your music."

That was good to hear. I had an intervention with her a couple of weeks earlier that left me wondering what she was thinking, especially about music therapy. She was pleasant and optimistic, but not talkative. In fact, when I had attempted to start a songwriting exercise with her, she verbally ended the session. After discussing the incident with the other music therapist, we decided that my approach with her wasn't quick or engaging enough. I was determined to try again with the knowledge that I'd gained from processing our last session.

This time, when I asked the patient to choose a song from the list, she said to her daughter, "Why don't you choose one." Her daughter said, "No, this is for you." I was ready to swoop in and suggest something, but before I did, the patient requested "How about, 'He's Got the Whole World in His Hands'? I was thrilled, because this song provides a good opportunity for easy lyric additions to help make the song more personal to the patient.

After a few verses, I said, "Who would you like to sing about? Any friends or family names you'd like to put into the song?"

"My whole family, I guess," she said. As we sang this verse, she smiled. She then asked for "Oh, What a Beautiful Morning." I sang the song through once and decided this would be the basis of our songwriting exercise. I quickly came up with a first line, "The sun's shining outside the window, oh, the sun's shining outside the window."

"What do you hear?" I asked. The patient said, "Noise," and laughed. I incorporated hospital noise into the next line asked if she had any ideas for the last line before the chorus. "I can choose another song," she said. To be honest, it shocked me. After four lines and some laughter, I still hadn't engaged her. I kept it going long enough to add in some lyrics about the end of her hospital stay, sang the chorus once, and ended the song. I was at a loss. I had failed to get the patient to open up in the session.

At this point, the other music therapist entered the room. She had her violin, which sparked some conversation. The patient's daughter said, "My mom used to play the violin."

The patient spoke about it for a short time. She had played many years ago in school. She didn't have the violin anymore, because she gave it to her granddaughter, who played it for a while and then gave it up. After this conversation, the patient chose another song. She smiled as the therapists sang and played.

I asked, "Would you like another song?" "No, thank you," she said, "That's all." She was a woman of few words. We thanked her and left the room.

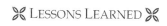

Some patients are difficult to assess. Some sessions remind me that I've learned a lot about being a music therapist. This one reminded me that learning is continuous.

PATIENCE IS A VIRTUE
Soothing an Agitated Client

I was in the lobby preparing to see a patient when a middle-aged man approached me and asked if we played music. He was interested in our instruments, especially the Q-Chord. He headed out of the lobby, and I gathered up my resources for session.

As I peered into the patient's room to check to see if he was still awake, the man who approached me told me that he was my patient's son-in-law and that he had been bringing his guitar and playing Bob Dylan music for him when he came to visit. I asked if I could spend some time with his father-in-law, but he looked hesitant and said, "I don't know if it's a good time. He is really agitated, and I don't know if it will help." I suggested trying one song to see if I could help the patient relax, and he agreed. I entered the room, introduced myself to the patient, and immediately noticed his agitation. He was moaning and his movements seemed stiff. I assured the patient that all he had to do was relax and listen.

I began finger picking at a slow tempo on the guitar and hummed the melody of "Edelweiss" and then "Shenandoah." I considered playing some Bob Dylan, but I wasn't sure if that was his music taste or that of his son-in-law. The patient was still agitated, and his son-in-law looked fidgety and doubtful. I asked if I could try one more, and he said, "Sure, but I don't think he can hear it." I reassured that the patient could still hear, even if he couldn't verbally respond. Another family friend entered the room, so I introduced myself while the son-in-law stepped outside for a moment.

✄ LESSONS LEARNED ✄

"It reminded me that sometimes I need to be more patient in waiting for outcomes."

I decided to try "Blowin' in the Wind," with guitar finger picking and vocal humming. The patient immediately relaxed, the moaning had stopped, and he was still. At one point, he fell asleep, but awoke again as I finished the song. The family friend said, "I am amazed. The music had such a calming effect. Thank you so much for what you do." The son-in-law returned, and he thanked me as well.

This was a great session because I had struggled in the past with clients who are physically agitated. Often in the hospital setting, I would play a couple of songs for similar patients and see no change. I usually give up after ten minutes, but sometimes I feel like I leave too early. I promised myself that next time I encountered an agitated client, I would stay a little longer and experiment with different finger picking and strumming patterns, in addition to singing and humming. I am glad that I stayed for one more song with this patient because I finally did see a positive effect.

FIRST IMPRESSIONS
Bringing Out the Best in Patients

On my second day bringing instruments to the cancer center, I facilitated two successful interventions right off the bat. After these, I went to the other side of the room and introduced myself to a few patients. One man I had met the day before, and from that encounter, I did not feel that he would want music therapy at all.

Today was a different story; he openly welcomed me. I asked the woman next to him if it was alright for me to play music, since she was watching a movie with headphones from her portable DVD player. She said the movie was over and music would be fine. After chatting a bit, the male client mentioned that although his wife had been a wonderful pianist, he was not a musician. In fact, he tried for three months after she passed away to learn, but he gave up. He did, however, sing second tenor in several choirs throughout his lifetime.

I asked him if he knew how to sing in harmony for a duet, to which he complied. He suggested "I've Been Working on the Railroad." It took me a while to figure out what keys were good for a male whose voice was that high, but through trial and error and much transposing, we made it. He had a difficult time finding harmonies and decided to sing along with the melody. We sang several songs together on the guitar. The woman next to us listened.

After a few songs, I told him it was time he learned an instrument, and I reached for the Q-Chord. I showed him the "keyboard" function, and then I showed him the "chord" function. I explained how the chords in the book corresponded to the music, and asked him to give it a try. We looked at "You are My Sunshine" and he found C, F, and G. He was amazed that he was making music. We sang the song while he played the chords. He wanted to go on, so I challenged him and showed him 7th chords. We did the song one more time, and he played it perfectly, letting out a sigh of relief when we finished. I left happy that day. My goal was for the patients to have a positive experience with music therapy, and they all were pleased.

✖ LESSONS LEARNED ✖

"I realized that talking about music therapy and doing it brings about totally different results."

I learned to just go for it. Many times I will believe what the patient thinks of their musical abilities instead of trusting that they can try it and succeed.

THIRD TIME IS A CHARM
A Man with Aphasia

While catching up on referrals, a nurse came up to me and said, "I have a patient who might want music therapy, but he is aphasic." I told her that he might be able to sing with me. She gave me the "Do you even know what aphasia means?" look.

When I entered the patient's room, the nurse was taking his vitals. She spoke to him and he grunted in response. When I asked if he would like music, he nodded his head "yes."

At first, I was hesitant to ask him to sing with me. I had never done something like this with a patient with aphasia. I thought, "Is it going to frustrate him if I ask him to sing with me? How far should I push it? What should I say?" So I told him that I realized it was difficult for him to communicate and may be frustrating when others ask him to do so, but that singing may actually help with that. He smiled and laughed. Although he didn't sing along, he shook the egg shaker excitedly throughout the song. "Let's try to sing this next one together," I said, trying to use fewer words to explain my request. Still nothing. But he laughed and had a good time.

Should I ask a third time? "Alright, let's sing this song together. I will sing the first part and then look at you to sing the other parts." I sang, "You are my..." "Su-shy," the patient responded. Yes! I was so excited. We sang the whole song through once together in this fashion. The second time through the song he sang all of the words to the first verse independently.

When I was walking by his room later, I overheard the nurse telling his wife that a music therapist came in and that he sang along with her. The nurse told his wife that he had a great time.

If at first you don't succeed, try again. If you still don't succeed, try it a different way and take a new approach. People continue to surprise me. A very fine line separates pushing too hard and giving up. Often, my timid nature comes off as "giving up." I don't want to step on toes. I am realizing that this is not the case for effective music therapy. To try new things and create new ideas, we must pursue our goals by walking that fine line.

ALL THE BELLS AND WHISTLES
Believe in the Capabilities of You and Your Client

I spotted a patient while I was doing cold rounds in the hospital, but the occupational therapists beat me to the room. As I returned from seeing another patient, I observed the occupational therapists struggling a bit with the same patient. They were trying to keep him awake and stimulated. I poked my head in the room, and they said excitedly, "Are you coming in here?" I explained I was planning to and could do so immediately if it would be useful. "Yes, please," replied the occupational therapist, "we're trying to keep him awake, and we want him to use his arms."

As my assessment and therapeutic wheels began to turn, I quickly reached for my songbook and drums. I held out the mallet to the patient, and asked the occupational therapists if he was right handed. They weren't sure, but he immediately used that hand to grasp the extended mallet. I directed the paddle drum to his left hand.

The patient began to strike the drum in a steady four beat pattern. I began to accompany him with "When the Saints Go Marching In." He focused on his playing with great concentration and followed my tempo as it fluctuated between a very fast to a moderate tempo. The occupational therapists stood amazed: "Oh, now you're going to wake up!" they laughed.

After several minutes of playing, I asked the patient if he recognized that song. Nothing. Then I waited 15 seconds or so, thinking I needed to let him process. He opened his mouth, smiled, and said, "Yes." The patient also participated by not only playing the jingle stick, but also exploring different ways to play it, including crossing his midline and tapping it on his opposite hand.

I was curious to see if I could get the patient to vocalize more and give him the opportunity to use his voice. I chose "Home on the Range." I sang through the first verse and chorus, and he stared at the tray in front of him. I went back to the top of the song, slower this time and slowed down the end of phrases. I said to him, "I want you to fill in the words. "Oh give me a...?" He glanced up a bit, "Home." I was amazed and kept going. "Where the buffalo..." "Roam!" he spoke even clearer this time and continued on singing whole phrases. At some parts, I dropped out my singing all together. By the end of the verse and chorus, he was smiling and singing louder than ever. I turned my head a bit toward the door and saw a few of the nurses in the station peeking from behind the counter. This was obviously a big deal for him. I said my goodbyes to the patient and told him I would be back. Music really reached him. I not only stimulated him and kept him awake, but I got real responses with music. I thought, "Don't judge a book by its cover. He was way more capable than I would have initially thought."

This was the first session I stepped out of my comfort zone and explored my music therapy skills tool belt. I realized I could think on my toes, get positive results, and help a patient show off all he is capable of accomplishing.

Chapter 12: Questions for growth

1. A perfect record is not always achievable in a hospital setting. What do you think is an appropriate ratio of declines verses approvals for your practice?

2. A lot of these excerpts deal with the therapist having a preconceived idea about how the way things might go in a session. Having an open mind about things is good, but when do you think it is appropriate to have a closed mind? Are there times when you should remain closed off to something?

3. Trusting in your own abilities as a music therapist can be hard at times, especially when you have to go with the flow. Here is some practice: You are doing a co-treat session with two patients in a room. One patient is mellow and needs to get up; one patient is anxious and needs to settle down. Using the isoprinciple, how do you treat these clients simultaneously considering where they are both at and where they need to get to through music therapy?

4. Many times in this chapter it has been mentioned, "patience is a virtue." Have you found yourself in a similar situation in your practicum or internship experiences?

5. As a therapist with clinical education we know the potential of the patients more than they often know. In "Third Time is a Charm," the therapist is asking

the patient to do something that is uncomfortable for him considering his diagnoses. Was asking him three times to participate too much?

6. Part of being able to successfully lead a client to fill-in-the-blanks of a song, is that you must be able to do it. Using the first example in this chapter of a fill-in-the-blank exercise, complete the following to the song, "The Rose."

Some say _____, it is _____,

_____.

Some say _____, it is _____,

_____.

Some say _____, it is _____,

_____.

I say _____, it is _____,

_____.

7. Take a look at the next two lessons learned: "If you don't try, you'll never know how successful something could be," and "As therapists, we're constantly learning and growing. It never stops." Reflect on these lessons personally as they may pertain to you and/or discuss these lessons learned in a group.

CONCLUSION

> "Remember, if you ever need a helping
> hand, it's at the end of your arm, as you
> get older, remember you have another
> hand: The first is to help yourself, the
> second is to help others."

> —Audrey Hepburn

I hope you have enjoyed reading *Six-Month Chrysalis*.
This book is more than a compilation of stories; it is filled
with confessions, taboo topics, and intimate moments of
that which we don't often get to express: client
experiences. Sometimes, putting the magical and/or
growing moments we experience in our ever-changing days
into words is difficult. This book acts as a qualitative
reflection of the interventions, processes, and outcomes we
observe; perhaps it will inspire you to collect your own
stories of music and humanity!

The use of this book is up to you: a handbook, a heart-
felt read, a conversation starter as it sits atop your coffee
table. If you are a student or current intern, I hope this
provides you with some insight into the world of an
intern. Although everyone's "chrysalis" is unique, this may
qualify as a powerful tool to reflect back to in times of joy
and struggle. For professionals, you may find yourself
remembering those moments when you were just a
"caterpillar" in the field. Internship supervisors can relearn
the perspective of an intern, and use these reflections to

grow as a mentor. For all of us, we can relate to the moments of human connection, joy and grief, and especially growth. We are always learning, expanding, and emerging as butterflies with beautiful music as our wings and therapy as our path to fly.

ABOUT THE ORGANIZER

Sarah R. Sendlbeck is an alumna of the MusicWorx clinical internship. Originally from Buffalo, New York, she moved to San Diego in June 2011 to complete her clinical internship. During this time, she worked with a variety of populations including general hospital, substance abuse and addiction, Parkinson's disease, military (post-traumatic stress disorder), bonding program for teen mothers and their infants, cancer support groups, pulmonary groups, hospice care, the homeless, adults with developmental disabilities, Rett syndrome, and female victims of trafficking and domestic violence.

Sarah received her Bachelors of Music in music therapy from Nazareth College of Rochester with a minor in psychology, and her Masters in Entrepreneurship from Oklahoma State University. Sarah is an innovator and is passionate about incorporating new technology while working with her patients. She spent three years working in hospice care throughout the city of Boston, while also teaching music, art, and drama at a Montessori school in the north shore. After having her daughter in 2015, Sarah has stepped away from client work to travel all over the United States with her family, focus on various passion projects, while raising her daughter.

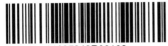

Made in the USA
Lexington, KY
15 October 2018